Rose's Strategy of Preventive Medicine

Rose's Strategy of Preventive Medicine

The complete original text

Geoffrey Rose

Emeritus Professor of Epidemiology,
London School of Hygiene and Tropical Medicine, UK

With a commentary by

Kay-Tee Khaw

Professor of Clinical Gerontology,
University of Cambridge, UK

Michael Marmot

Professor of Epidemiology,
University College London, UK

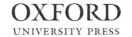

UNIVERSITY PRESS

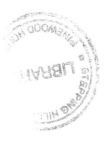

OXFORD

UNIVERSITY PRESS

Great Clarendon Street, Oxford OX2 6DP

Oxford University Press is a department of the University of Oxford.
It furthers the University's objective of excellence in research, scholarship,
and education by publishing worldwide in

Oxford New York

Auckland Cape Town Dar es Salaam Hong Kong Karachi
Kuala Lumpur Madrid Melbourne Mexico City Nairobi
New Delhi Shanghai Taipei Toronto

With offices in

Argentina Austria Brazil Chile Czech Republic France Greece
Guatemala Hungary Italy Japan Poland Portugal Singapore
South Korea Switzerland Thailand Turkey Ukraine Vietnam

Published in the United States by Oxford University Press Inc., New York
in the UK and in certain other countries

Published in the United States
by Oxford University Press Inc., New York

A catalogue record for this book is available from the British Library
Library of Congress Cataloging in Publication Data

Data available

Typeset by Cepha Imaging Private Ltd., Bangalore, India
Printed in Great Britain
on acid-free paper by
Clays Ltd., Bungay, Suffolk, UK

ISBN 978–0–19–263097–1

10 9 8 7 6 5 4 3 2 1

Whilst every effort has been made to ensure that the contents of this book are as
complete, accurate and-up-to-date as possible at the date of writing. Oxford
University Press is not able to give any guarantee or assurance that such is the case.
Readers are urged to take appropriately qualified medical advice in all cases. The
information in this book is intended to be useful to the general reader, but should
not be used as a means of self-diagnosis or for the prescription of medication.

Preface

Geoffrey Rose was a key figure in the enormous progress that has been made worldwide in the last few decades in the epidemiology and prevention of cardiovascular disease. His work spanned the first studies identifying risk factors for coronary heart disease in individuals ('Why did this individual get this disease?'), epidemiological studies examining the occurrence of coronary heart disease in populations ('Why does this population have so much disease?'), intervention trials ('Can we prevent coronary heart disease and stroke?') and ultimately, the development and of preventive clinical practice and public health policy ('What should we do to reduce coronary heart disease and stroke ocurrence in individuals and populations?'). However, his influence extends far beyond cardiovascular disease. By improving both the practical and theoretical scientific tools of epidemiologic investigation he fostered advancements in the entire field. Ultimately, his insights into the relationship between ill health, or deviance, in individuals and the populations they come from, have changed our whole approach to strategies for improving the health, in its broadest sense, of individuals and populations.

Geoffrey Rose was a Scholar both at Queen's College, Oxford and then at St Mary's Hospital Medical School, London, qualifying in medicine in 1949. He subsequently held clinical posts at St Mary's Hospital where he began his lifelong interest in the treatment and prevention of cardiovascular disease. He joined the research staff of the London School of Hygiene and Tropical Medicine in 1959, becoming Lecturer, then Reader in Epidemiology there before returning to St Mary's as Professor of Epidemiology in 1970. In 1977 he was appointed Professor of Epidemiology at the London School of Tropical Medicine and Hygiene. Through his whole professional career he continued his clinical work at St Mary's Hospital. Indeed, the bridging of clinical medicine, with its focus on individuals, and epidemiology and public health, with their focus on populations, was a constant theme throughout his life.

One of Geoffrey Rose's concerns both as a clinician and scientist was that inferences are only as good as the data on which they are based. When he started research work in the 1960s, there were no generally accepted standardized methods for diagnosis of coronary heart disease in populations and his initial work focused on developing more valid measurement methods. These included an early prototype for the random zero sphygmomanometer for measurement of blood pressure, the Rose Cardiovascular questionnaire, and, with an American colleague, Henry Blackburn, the Minnesota Code for the classification of electrocardiographic abnormalities. The manual he prepared in 1968 with Henry Blackburn, for the World Health Organization, *Cardiovascular Survey Methods*, is still the international standard.

He chaired numerous national and international committees including the Medical Research Council Hypertension Trial Working Party and the MRC Neural Tube Defect Trial Steering Committees, and the World Health Organization Expert Committees on Prevention of Coronary Heart Disease. His research contributions were prolific: the Whitehall Study of London civil servants and the WHO European Collaborative Trial of Coronary Heart Disease, encompassing centres in Belgium, Italy, Poland, Spain and UK are just two examples of studies among the many he led which contributed greatly to the understanding of the causes and prevention of coronary heart disease.

However, it was the INTERSALT study—an international co-operative study of blood pressure patterns and their determinants in 52 communities, that led to his most fundamental appraisal of the relationship between ill health in individuals and ill health in populations. In his earlier writings he noted that medical practice is largely concerned with treating sick individuals. However,

a rescue operation of this nature may be entirely appropriate, but it can no more solve the problem of mass diseases than famine relief can solve the problem of hunger in the Third World . . . The radical solution is to identify and if possible to remedy the underlying causes of our major health problems.

(Rose 1992)

During his early clinical training with Sir George Pickering at St Mary's he received the notion that a population can be studied as an entity, for between its extremists (the sick) and its masses (normal people) there exists a continuity: people who are hypertensives are simply the tail end of a normal distribution. Hence, apparently individual clinical problems such as heart attacks are part of a problem in the whole community. The INTERSALT study demonstrated that the proportion of persons who were defined as 'hypertensive' was directly related to the population mean level of blood pressure. The same finding applied to behavioural factors such as alcohol intake, that is, the proportion of high alcohol drinkers was directly related to the population level of alcohol. Thus, the sick:

hypertensives, the alcoholics . . . represent simply the extreme of a continuous distribution of risk or behaviour. When different populations are compared, the distribution is seen to shift up or down as a coherent whole. The essential determinants of the health of society are thus to be found in its mass characteristics: the deviant minority can only be understood when seen in its societal context, and effective prevention requires changes which involve the population as a whole.

(Rose 1992)

Geoffrey Rose saw teaching as inextricably linked to his work as clinician and scientist and in this, as in all his other roles, he was outstanding. The clarity and originality which characterized his thinking was reflected in his writing and lecturing. His articles and lectures were always a model of precision and brevity; his ideas were never cluttered with extraneous material. He was responsible for training whole generations of epidemiologists not just in Britain but internationally. In 1968, together with colleagues Richard Remington and Rose and Jerry Stamler from the United States, he initiated the annual International Society and Federation of Cardiology Ten Day Teaching Seminars in Cardiovascular Disease Prevention and Epidemiology. The aim was to strengthen efforts to prevent mass cardiovascular disease by providing training to physicians and scientists around the world. These seminars have now been taking place for 40 years, and have trained over 1200 people from over 100 nations in the aetiology and prevention of cardiovascular disease. For many, the seminar transformed the direction of their professional and scientific lives. The majority of the current international leaders in the field of cardiovascular epidemiology are former fellows of the 10-day seminars. However, a no less important aim of the seminar, which reflected the humanitarian concerns of Geoffrey Rose and his colleagues, was the breaking down of barriers and making bridges across countries and cultures through peaceful international scientific co-operation. Many past fellows have stressed that the seminar has been most inspiring not only in terms of academic goals but in terms of personal friendships made and mutual trust engendered. This was exemplified by the INTERSALT study. The 52 different communities studied included Yanomano and Xingu from Brazil, Luo from Kenya, and groups from countries such as Papua New Guinea, Japan, the People's Republic of China, the former German Democratic Republic, the former Soviet Union, United States, and Trinidad and Tobago. This was a unique example of how despite the diversity of background and cultures of the several hundred scientific collaborators it was possible to resolve differences and work together, using a standard agreed protocol, towards a common scientific goal.

Geoffrey Rose's personal qualities were of course an integral part of his success as a clinician, scientist and teacher. There are few people in whom the qualities of kindness and devastating honesty and integrity can coexist without contradiction: when asked for an opinion, he could always be relied on to tell the truth, which was sometimes painful, but this was always done with such thoughtfulness and concern that lessons were taken on board. Similarly, he combined the qualities of scientific scepticism, recognizing that data are subject to error and therefore theories are impermanent and liable to be superseded, with a deep faith in the inherent goodness of people. He brought out the best in everyone by simply believing in and expecting the best from them.

Research findings are deemed outstanding if they last a decade. Clinical results are even more fleeting. However, for numberless students and professional colleagues worldwide the impact Geoffrey Rose had on their lives was profound and permanent. His scientific and humanitarian ideals and personal example caused many to approach life and learning in a different way and in turn to influence others.

The strength and calm which emanated from Geoffrey Rose derived from his steadfast religious faith, as well his harmonious family life, in particular, his exceptionally happy marriage to Ceridwen and their two sons and daughter.

Both of us had the immense privilege of being taught by, and working with, Geoffrey Rose. There is something very special about having been a student or colleague of Geoffrey's. Throughout the world, we have had this extraordinary experience of meeting strangers at scientific meetings and recognizing the common bond of having shared the same transforming experience.

When Geoffrey asked us to take on further editions of his book, it was evident that the clarity of his voice and ideas still hold and did not need updating and elaboration. His ideas have influenced many in innumerable ways. Our commentary simply is a brief reflection of our personal perspectives.

Kay-Tee Khaw
Michael Marmot

Preface adapted from an obituary for Geoffrey Rose published in the *Times* on November 12, 1993.

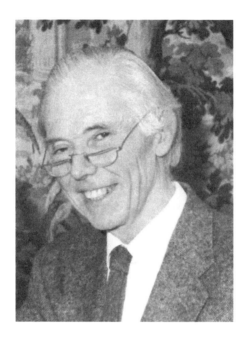

Geoffrey Rose, CBE, physician and epidemiologist, Emeritus Professor of Epidemiology, London School of Hygiene and Tropical Medicine and Honorary Consultant Physician, St. Mary's Hospital Medical School, London was born on April 19, 1926 and died on November 12, 1993 aged 67.

We are all responsible to all for all

DOSTOEVSKY, *The Brothers Karamazov*

Preface to the original edition

Medical thinking has been largely concerned with responding to the needs of sick individuals. This has shaped its ethics (responsibility for the sick), its research questions ('Why do individuals become sick?'), and the planning of services (a response to demand from patient-initiated consultations). This thinking has now been extended into risk identification and disease prevention: general practitioners seek out individuals with hypertension, occupational physicians try to ensure that no one is exposed to an excess of a toxic substance, and medical concern about alcohol is focused on the 'problem drinkers'.

The aim of all these endeavours is to help a vulnerable minority of individuals. A rescue operation of this nature may be entirely appropriate, but it can no more solve the problem of mass diseases than famine relief can solve the problem of hunger in the Third World. The strategy is symptomatic, not radical.

The radical strategy is to identify and if possible to remedy the underlying causes of our major health problems. It then commonly emerges that those whom we particularly wish to help, such as the hypertensives, the alcoholics, and others with special problems, represent simply the extreme of a continuous distribution of risk or behaviour; when different populations are compared, the distribution is seen to shift up or down as a coherent whole. The essential determinants of the health of society are thus to be found in its mass characteristics: the deviant minority can only be understood when seen in its societal context, and effective prevention requires changes which involve the population as a whole.

The purpose of this book is to examine, with diverse examples, the various strategies of prevention, each with its strengths and limitations, and to explore, more fully than has previously been attempted, the often disturbing implications for policy, research, and ethics of the population-wide approach to the prevention of common medical and behavioural disorders. The health of society is integral, and the supposedly 'normal' majority needs to accept responsibility for its deviant minority—however loth it may be to do so.

Geoffrey Rose
1992

Acknowledgements from the original edition

It is appropriate that this book should start, as it will continue, by acknowledging that individuals belong to a society. One individual's thoughts do not spring fully formed from the mind's womb, rather we receive from others, then if the times are favourable we enhance or augment, and we hand on to our successors. From my teacher, Professor Sir George Pickering, I received the notion that a population can be studied as an entity, for between its extremists ('the sick') and its masses ('normal people') there exists a continuity. Later, from the work of Professor Ancel Keys I caught the idea that there are healthy populations and there are sick populations. All else that appears in this book is simply an outworking of these two notions.

To give formal expression to ideas calls for a secretary, and none could have served me more loyally or effectively than Mrs Susan Teoh. Over a period of many years Miss Linda Colwell and Martin Shipley have supplied me with trustworthy data. Finally, for detecting some of the book's falsities and rough corners I am indebted to my friends and critics, Professors David Barker, Nicholas Wald, and W.R. Ward, and Dr Derek Middleton.

Contents

Commentary

Kay-Tee Khaw and Michael Marmot

Introduction

Geoffrey Rose's insights into the inextricable relationship between ill health, or deviance, in individuals and the populations from which they come have changed our whole approach to strategies for improving health, in its broadest sense, of individuals and populations. The concepts underlying the strategy of preventive medicine, and the high-risk and population approach are now so widely accepted that it is hard to realize how radical they were when first outlined. These ideas were first published in his seminal articles in the 1980s and brought together in his book, *The Strategy of Preventive Medicine*, in 1992. The book describes with characteristic clarity, succinctness, and coherence the population distribution as the central focus in thinking about prevention. The clear vision and voice of Geoffrey speaks in this book.

However, two decades after his ideas were first published, during which the human genome project and other major scientific advances such as gene therapy have promised to transform our approach to treatment and health care with the emphasis on personalized medicine, we believe Rose's ideas still have currency and relevance, and his ideas about population-level characteristics need to continue to inform our strategies for improving health.

The Rose concepts and applications

Geoffrey Rose started out as a clinician interested in the epidemic of cardiovascular disease and what best could be done not just to treat but to prevent the disease. He began with the usual clinical question of why a particular individual developed disease. He was part of a movement that sought to identify what could be done to prevent disease by identifying causal pathways. This is now standard fare, but, at the time, it was an important innovation to identify factors that increased risk of heart disease, such as raised blood pressure and raised blood lipids.

An important conceptual shift came with the realization that risk and disease are a continuum in the population; virtually all pathophysiological factors examined were continuously distributed in the population, and high risk and sick individuals simply represent the extreme end of a distribution. Early approaches to prevention by screening to identify those at very high risk of disease, essentially an extension of the clinical model, required understanding of how risk factors were distributed in the population and how they related to the disease.

This led to the next major insight that the total burden of disease in a community depended on the numbers of people exposed to a particular risk factor, i.e. the population distribution of a risk factor. A large number of people in the centre of the distribution, exposed to small elevations in risk, contribute more cases to a population than a small number of people at the extreme of the distribution exposed to a very high risk. Thus, prevention of cardiovascular disease needed to consider not just screening and treatment in those at very high risk at the extremes of the distribution, the 'high-risk strategy', but reduction of risk factors in the large numbers of those in the middle of the distribution with moderately elevated risk, the 'mass population strategy'.

Rose also realized that as with risk, the definition of disease in a population was to some extent arbitrary; individuals with overt symptomatic coronary disease, for example, were at one extreme end of a spectrum in the population of people with none, or varying degrees of coronary atherosclerosis, often asymptomatic. The extension of this single population distribution model from risk of disease to disease itself was described in his analyses of data from the Intersalt study. If individuals who had a disease were simply those at the extreme of a population distribution, then the prevalence of disease in any given population, i.e. the number of individuals who cross some defining threshold, is directly related to where the population distribution is located on an absolute scale, as reflected by the population mean. The causes of individual cases (i.e. what determines differences between individuals who do and do not get disease in a particular population or their position in the population distribution) are not necessarily the same as the causes of disease incidence, i.e. the position of the population distribution as a whole, which determines the number of individuals who fall outside any particular absolute threshold. Thus, prevention strategies, to be effective, would not just focus on the high-risk individuals at one extreme of the distribution, but would have to address the population distribution.

Continuity of risk and population impact

The continuous relationship between level of blood pressure and cholesterol and risk of cardiovascular disease, documented extensively in numerous population studies, is now widely accepted to the extent that risk is now recognized as a continuum in the population. Thus, those at high risk are just one extreme of the distribution and, as Rose noted, definitions of high risk are generally arbitrary though necessary for clinical action. Decisions to screen for risk and to treat are moving towards criteria based on quantitative assessment of absolute risk and judgements about risk–benefit and cost–benefit balances. The numerous cardiovascular risk charts now in use estimating absolute cardiovascular disease risk for different groups stratified by age, sex, and risk factor levels recognize the continuum of risk (De Backer *et al.* 2003). It is also increasingly evident that this continuous relationship between level of risk factor and risk of cardiovascular disease applies to the many new risk factors for cardiovascular disease including inflammatory markers such as C-reactive protein and glycated haemoglobin (Khaw *et al.* 2004*a*), an indicator of glucose metabolism.

Examples: intraocular pressure and glaucoma; bone health and fractures
The continuum of risk between a risk factor and disease is now recognized for many disparate conditions such as raised intraocular pressure and incidence of open angle glaucoma (Leske et al. 2002), or bone density measures (Khaw *et al.* 2004*a*) and subsequent fracture risk, as illustrated in Fig. 1(a–c), and has led to the development of similar absolute risk assessment approaches for glaucoma and fracture incorporating several risk factors to enable identification of individuals at greatest absolute risk who would most benefit from preventive interventions (Fechtner and Khouri 2007; Kanis *et al.* 2007).

A large number of people at small risk may give rise to more cases of disease than a small number of people at high risk

The further dimension that Rose highlighted is that though it is possible to focus our preventive efforts on very high-risk groups, these are a relatively small proportion of the population.

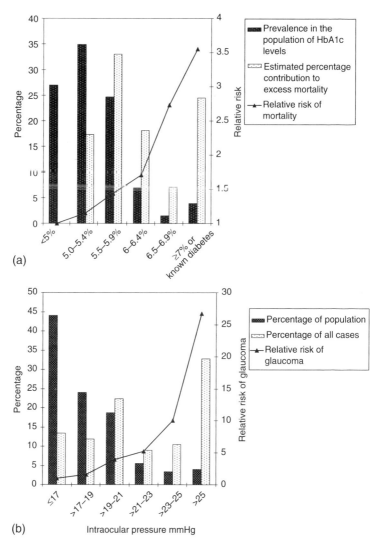

Fig. 1 (a) Distribution of glycated haemoglobin (HbA1c) concentrations in men and women aged 45–79 years, relative risk of mortality by HbA1c, and estimated percentage contribution to excess mortality at different levels of HbA1c (Khaw *et al.* 2004a). (b) Distribution of intraocular pressure in the Barbados Eye Study, relative risk of open angle glaucoma, and distribution of glaucoma cases in the population at different levels of intraocular pressure (Leske *et al.* 2002).

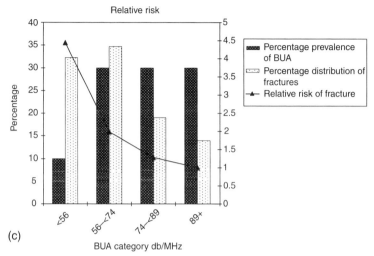

(c)

Fig.1 (*Cont.*) (c) Distribution of bone heel ultrasound (BUA) measures in men and women aged 42–82 years, relative risk of incident fractures, and percentage of fractures occurring in the population by bone by BUA measure (Khaw *et al.* 2004*b*).

Examples: intraocular pressure and glaucoma; bone health and fractures; cardiovascular disease As Fig. 1(a–c) also illustrates, the majority of cases in the population occur not in the small numbers at very high risk but in the centre of the population distribution, where large numbers of people are exposed, albeit with only modest increases in risk. Thus, as can be seen in the various examples, even though intraocular pressure levels above 25 mmHg are associated with nearly 25-fold increased risk of glaucoma, the 4 per cent of the population who have these levels contribute about a third of the cases and the other two-thirds occur in the larger numbers who are at moderately elevated risk. Similarly, while about 30 per cent of the fractures in the population occur in the 10 per cent of the population with low bone density measured by bone heel ultrasound attenuation (BUA), 70 per cent of the fractures occur in the rest of the population.

Thus, efforts to prevent disease aimed at screening and treatment of individuals at very high risk are likely to have only limited population impact, as the majority of cases would not occur in the very high-risk group. Rose suggested that a complement to the high-risk strategy would be shifting the whole population distribution of a risk factor. As Tables 1 and 2 show, relatively small reductions in the population distribution of cardiovascular disease risk factors (Emberson *et al.* 2004) or bone health (Khaw *et al.* 2004*b*) might be estimated to have an impact in the population similar to or greater than an approach which targeted those at high risk.

The theoretical estimates have been largely supported by analyses examining changes in cardiovascular disease rates in different countries. One report examining the observed halving of age-adjusted

Table 1 A comparison of approaches to the primary prevention of cardiovascular disease based on data from the British Regional Heart Study (Emberson *et al.* 2004).

'High-risk' approach	Management	RRR (%)	Framingham 10-year CHD event risk		
			≥40%	≥20%	≥15%
Treatment decision based on overall absolute risk	Statin	30	5%	15%	21%
	Beta-blocker/ diuretic	22	4%	11%	16%
	Aspirin, statin, ACE inhibitor, and beta-blocker/diuretic	68	11%	34%	59%
Population 'shifting mean' approach			**'Shift' the risk factor distribution by**		
			5%	**10%**	**15%**
Reduce cholesterol in the population			12%	22%	32%
Reduce systolic blood pressure			16%	29%	40%
Reduce both mean cholesterol and systolic blood pressure			26%	45%	59%

RRR = relative risk reduction: the percentage reduction in cardiovascular disease expected with use of the intervention.

Table 2 Estimated population impact of high-risk and 'shifting mean' approach to bone heel ultrasound attenuation (BUA) on fractures (Khaw *et al.* 2004*b*).

Estimated population reduction in fractures with treatment of those with lowest 10% of BUA distribution and fracture risk halved	16%
Estimated population reduction in fractures if mean BUA increased by 0.25 standard deviation	14%
Estimated population reduction in fractures if mean BUA increased by 0.5 standard deviation	23%

mortality rates for coronary heart disease in US deaths 1980–2000 estimated that approximately half the decline could be attributable to reductions in major risk factors in the general population and half to evidence-based medical therapies. Similar analyses for other countries such as The Netherlands and Finland give comparable or higher estimates for the impact of changes in risk factor distributions (Ford *et al.* 2007).

This has led to the impetus to identify the environmental or lifestyle factors such as diet or physical activity that may influence the population distribution of risk factors.

The population mean predicts the prevalence of cases

While the mass population approach to prevention by shifting the population distribution of risk factor has been widely discussed, particularly for cardiovascular disease, the more profound implications of this concept in wider areas have yet to be widely debated.

In analyses from the Intersalt study, Rose not only demonstrated that the prevalence of hypertension and obesity, using absolute cutoff point definitions, in 52 different and disparate populations worldwide were directly and highly correlated with the mean or median of each of those populations, but that this also applied to apparent behavioural variables such as alcohol intake.

His interpretation was that 'the essential determinants of the health of society are thus to be found in its mass characteristics: the deviant minority can only be understood when seen in its societal context, and effective prevention requires changes which involve the population as a whole'.

Rose reported further examples from mental health between prevalence of psychiatric morbidity and mean general population mental health scores (Anderson *et al.* 1993). Other examples have followed. Batchelor and Sheiham (2002) showed both in the USA and in Britain that the prevalence of dental caries was positively related to the mean dental health score in different communities, with an estimated increase of about 20 per cent in caries prevalence for every 0.5 unit increase in DMFT (decayed, missing, and filled teeth score). They concluded that the secular decline in prevalence of caries seen in both countries occurred throughout the population and was not confined to subgroups.

The reference to the health of society indicated Rose's thinking on issues beyond disease to extend to behavioural and other outcomes related to the health of society. If this principle holds, then factors which shift societal norms would be predicted also to relate to the prevalence of the related behavioural extremes. For example, one could postulate, as Rose did, relationships between mean alcohol intake and prevalence of alcoholism, gambling habits and problem gambling, depression and suicide rates, aggression and violent crime, etc. There is now increasing empirical support from a wide range of disparate examples. Where this takes us in terms of implications for policy is more difficult.

Example: gambling Grun and McKeigue (2000) have shown both secular and geographic relationships between mean or median household expenditure on gambling and the prevalence of problem gambling.

Household gambling expenditure in the UK was examined using Family Expenditure Survey data collected before and after the introduction of a national lottery in November 1994. In cross-sectional analyses, the mean or median household expenditure on gambling for each region in the UK predicted the prevalence of excessive gambling in that region: the slope of the relationship in 1995–1996 was equivalent to an increase in approximately 1 per cent in the percentage of households gambling more than 10 per cent of income for

Table 3 Relationship of proportion of households gambling excessively to average gambling expenditure by UK region, 1993–94 (before the National Lottery) and 1995–96 (after the National Lottery).

	Year	Regression coefficient (95% CI) of percentage of households per £1 increase in gambling expenditure
Percentage gambling > £20/week	1993–94	0.8 (0.5–1.0)
	1995–96	1.6 (1.1–2.1)
Percentage gambling > 10% income	1993–94	0.5 (0.1–0.8)
	1995–96	1.2 (0.7–1.7)

every increase of £1 in mean household gambling expenditure (Table 3). When average spending on gambling was doubled by the introduction of the National Lottery in the UK, there was a fourfold increase in the proportion of households where gambling expenditure was excessive. Among households with income of less than £200 per week, the proportion gambling more than 10 per cent of their income increased over fivefold (Grun and McKeigue 2000).

The direct relationship between the population mean and excessive gambling both geographically and over time led them to conclude that the single distribution theory applies to gambling behaviour: they suggested that measures to control deviance, the tail of a distribution, will have limited success if the entire distribution is shifting in the direction of the tail; thus any measures that increase the average level of gambling will increase the prevalence of excessive gambling and gambling disorders.

Between 2001 and 2005 the amount spent on gambling in the UK increased fourfold. The prediction is that the liberalization of gambling controls, such as with the Gaming Act in UK 2005 and the introduction in the UK of casinos and on line betting, is likely to shift population norms even further and result in a greatly increased prevalence of problem gambling.

Example: educational attainment Gambling and excessive alcohol intake might be considered as examples of social deviance and behavioural extremes analogous to the illness model. However, the single distribution model might also be applied to positive attributes at the opposite end of the distribution, such as academic attainment.

In educational attainment, the Trends in International Mathematics and Science Study (TIMSS) 2003 survey in 46 countries for students aged 14 (Mullis *et al.* 2004), the mean score for each country is directly related to the prevalence of those with high attainment and inversely related to the prevalence of those with poor attainment. A small difference in the mean of about a quarter of a standard deviation is associated with about a 5 per cent increase in the prevalence of high achievers and a 6 per cent decrease in the prevalence of those with poor attainment (Table 4). Despite the hugely differing cultural and educational systems internationally, the distribution of attainment in each country seems to be shifted up and down as a whole on an absolute scale. These differences are not genetic as distributions

Table 4 The association between prevalence of high and low achievers and the mean score in 46 different countries for mathematics and science at age 14 in Third International Maths and Science Survey 2003 (Mullis *et al.* 2004).

	Prevalence range	Regression slope beta (95% CI) for change in prevalence for an increase in mean score of 20 (about 0.25 standard deviation)
Mathematics		
(Mean score 467, SD 76, range of mean score 264–603)		
High achievers (score >550)	0–77%	+4.8%
Low achievers (score <400)	1–91%	−6.3%
Science		
(Mean score 471, SD 74, range of mean score 244–578)		
High achievers (score >550)	0–66%	+4.9%
Low achievers (score <400)	1–87%	−6.0%

and scores in different countries in surveys in the past decades have changed. There is no evidence from this study that some countries may have satisfactory achievement at high levels, but a 'long tail' at the bottom end, or vice versa.

Figure 2 shows the distribution of scores for mathematics for 46 countries and Fig. 3(a) and (b) the strong correlation between population mean scores and the prevalence of high and low attainment.

Much educational policy is geared towards extremes of the distributions, whether the tail end of the distribution, to identify failing groups, or focusing on those at the very top. However, the Rose population distribution model would suggest that while remedial measures may be necessary, in the longer term the only way is to improve the norm. Indeed, the secular changes in different directions in different countries indicate that the countries which showed the greatest improvements in reducing the prevalence of low achievers or increasing the prevalence of high achievers in education were those in which the norms or median scores changed the most.

Does this also apply to sporting prowess? We might predict that the likelihood of having sports champions at the very highest level depends on having higher population norms in that sport through many people being encouraged to participate rather than policies simply trying to focus efforts on established high achievers.

We might speculate further that the prevalence of people with high attainment in any field, whether artistic, scientific, or commercial, might relate to the population norms in those domains. Thus, efforts to improve the quality of scientific research or artistic endeavour in a country by focusing resources only on a small elite at the extreme top end may, as in the high-risk analogy, provide some short-term success, but ultimately are unlikely to have any lasting effect unless there is more widespread improvement of population standards.

Causes of population incidence and individual cases are not the same

The strong relationship between the prevalence of cases and the population mean led to the observation that the causes of population incidence and individual cases are not the same. This distinction is crucial when considering the role of genetics and individual susceptibility.

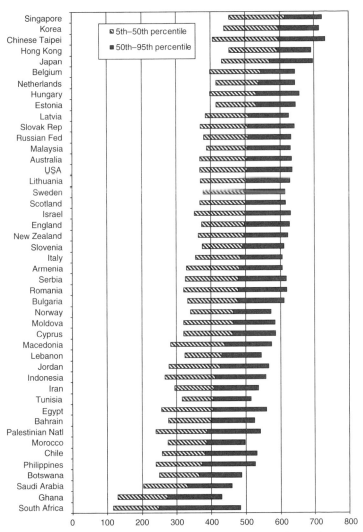

Fig. 2 Distribution of 5th, 50th, and 95th percentile scores for mathematics in 46 countries in the Trends in International Mathematics and Science 2003. Data from Mullis *et al.* (2004).

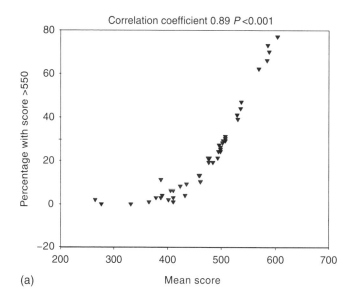

(a)

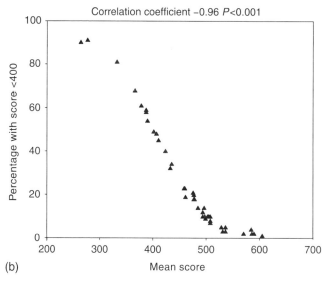

(b)

Fig. 3 (a) Correlation between prevalence of high achievers (score >550) in mathematics and mean score in 46 countries at age 14 (Mullis *et al.* 2004). Correlation coefficient 0.89, *P* <0.001. (b) Correlation between prevalence of low achievers (score <400) in mathematics and mean score in 46 countries at age 14 (Mullis *et al.* 2004). Correlation coefficient −0.96, *P* <0.001.

Genes and the genomic revolution

The human genome project has transformed our ability to identify the genes related to diseases, leading to speculation that in the future it will be possible to profile individuals for disease risk, and individuals can all have tailored interventions appropriate for their genetic profile. In the era of individualized medicine, do Rose's ideas still have relevance?

Though Rose's ideas pre-dated the human genome project, he recognized the advances in our understanding of genetic determinants and the increasing pre-eminence of genetic susceptibility which were easily encompassed and not incompatible with the population approach. The questions that are the focus of genetic profiling, i.e. the explanation of differences between individuals, are different from the questions that the population strategy addresses, that of explaining differences between populations. Indeed, focusing the question at the population level enables us to take most interesting aspects of the genetic technological advances and understanding further to ask the question of why there are such variations in gene expression and what the influences might be. Variants in specific genes have been associated with increased risk: recently, a common variant in the FTO gene present in 16 per cent was reported to be associated with body mass index and predisposes to childhood and adult obesity, with a 1.7-fold increased risk of obesity (Frayling *et al.* 2007). It is nevertheless evident that while the genetic profile may make some individuals more susceptible than others, i.e. why individuals may be at different ends of the spectrum, a different question, supported by major time trends and migration studies, is why populations with the same genetic profile have such different disease rates in different environments. The huge secular trends in increasing obesity witnessed in most countries (Mokdad *et al.* 1999) are not due to changing genetic profiles but changing behaviours.

A person with a genetic susceptibility may not develop disease in an environment where they are not exposed to whatever factors may influence gene expression. The challenge therefore, just as Geoffrey Rose pointed out, is to identify what the factors are that influence overall exposure in the population to shift the distribution and, thus, the numbers of those genetically susceptible who fall over the disease threshold. The ability to identify genetic susceptibility re-emphasizes the much greater challenge of assessing the environment and interactions with genes.

The clarification of the differences between individual and population risk also clarifies the confusion in the argument over the bell-shaped curve for intelligence. The argument that intelligence may have genetic influences (with which few people would disagree) has been fallaciously transposed to the proposition that the differences in distribution of intelligence test scores between different communities classified by social class or race are also attributable to genetic differences. However, the determinants of the population distribution location may be, and usually are, different from the determinants of interindividual differences within a population. Population distributions for variables such as intelligence test scores, obesity, cholesterol, and blood pressure vary enormously in different situations and reflect prevailing environmental and cultural norms.

If we compare different populations or even the same population over time, the population distribution shifts up and down on an absolute scale, such that the percentage of individuals who cross a particular threshold for disease varies depending on the placing of the population distribution. Thus, the major factors that determine why a particular individual develops a condition compared with others in the same population, i.e. the placing of the individual in a distribution, are not necessarily the same as the major factors that determine the placing of the population distribution as a whole, and hence why so many individuals in a particular population cross a threshold and develop the condition. Which aetiological factors appear to be important will be dependent on the homogeneity or heterogeneity of these factors within and between populations.

This brings the question back again to population and societal characteristics.

Societal characteristics

Consider these three statements:

1. In populations where mean plasma cholesterol levels are high, a great many people have raised levels of plasma cholesterol and the rate of coronary heart disease tends to be high.

2. If enough people in a closed community are immune to measles there will be herd immunity such that an individual with no immunity will have low probability of getting measles.

3. Populations characterized by high levels of social capital have lower rates of illness than those with low levels of social capital.

Each of these three requires us to go beyond the level of the individual in seeking the causes of the frequency of disease in populations. They operate in somewhat different ways, but they have in common the recognition that causes act at a population level.

In the first case we acknowledge that raised plasma cholesterol is a cause of coronary heart disease, but one of Rose's key insights was that the population average predicts the frequency of deviants. In this case, the mean cholesterol level of the population is a reasonable predictor of the proportion of people with raised cholesterol level. A second insight, which underlay the prevention paradox, was that the bulk of disease attributed to an exposure such as plasma cholesterol comes from the large mass of the population with moderate increases in the level of the risk factor, and a modest increase in relative risk of disease, as distinct from the small proportion with high levels of the risk factor and a large increase in relative risk. These two insights argue for looking at the causes of the distribution of risk factor levels—the causes of the causes. This is not problematic conceptually. If the nature of the fat content of the diet has an important influence on the plasma cholesterol distribution of the population, it is insufficient to focus, solely, on high-risk individuals. We need to inquire after the causes of the dietary pattern of the population. Characteristics such as custom, the operation of markets that affect supply, and hence price, promotion, and convenience will all be influences on the level of plasma cholesterol of individuals and hence the population distribution of plasma cholesterol.

This is not difficult conceptually. There are issues about the policy implications to which we will return. We can anticipate some of the problems raised by remembering that we applied Rose's single population theory not only to behaviours such as smoking and drinking but also to characteristics, such as gambling, that we do not associate directly with health.

The second case implies that there are characteristics of populations that derive from the properties of individuals, but that are true population-level characteristics. In the case of cholesterol, the mean population cholesterol is a simple arithmetic average of the individual cholesterol levels. An individual's risk is determined by his own cholesterol level, and the population level of disease risk is an average of the individual disease risks. We require a societal perspective when we think about improving things or, unhappily, recognizing why they are getting worse.

Not so in the case of herd immunity. The effect of an individual's immune status on his disease risk is dependent on the immune status of those around him. If enough people are immune in the closed community, then the number of susceptibles is too low to sustain transmission of the infectious agent. The non-immune individual is, therefore, at low risk because of a community-level characteristic—the level of herd immunity. This is almost the converse of the cholesterol example. It is not the individual's 'risk' status that determines his individual risk. Nor, indeed, is the level of population risk a simple sum of individual risks, although the number of immune individuals contributes, in a non-linear way, to the population level of risk. To restate: there is a societal level characteristic, herd immunity, that is derived from individual risks but can be considered an emergent property of the society.

This is familiar in the social sciences. Thomas Schelling won a Nobel Prize in economics for his contributions in bringing game theory into the economics of everyday life. In Schelling's view, game theory simply means that the behaviour of individuals is influenced by the behaviour of others (Schelling 1978). One of Schelling's examples is neighbourhood composition in the USA. He shows that racial segregation of neighbourhoods may not be the result of rampant racial prejudice. If each individual had a small predisposition to prefer living near people who were like them and hence a small tendency to move away when that was no longer the case, this could, in time, lead to neighbourhoods that tended towards complete racial segregation. Simply, if a small number of people of the 'other' group move in, a small number of people whose preference for homogeneity is a bit stronger than average will move out. A few more people move in and, as a result, a few more of the original residents move out. Note, that their preference for homogeneity may be weaker than that of the original outmigrants. This process can continue until the neighbourhood 'tips'. It then rapidly becomes homogeneous for the new group as the remainder of the original residents, whose preference for living next to people like them may only have been slight, then move away.

In the US context, racial issues become bound up with socioeconomic ones. What we may then observe is a neighbourhood whose socioeconomic character has shown a marked downturn. If the local tax base is now lower, schools will be inadequately funded, and other amenities and services will be lacking. These neighbourhood characteristics will, as discussed in our third example below, have an important effect on health. Remember, this societal-level characteristic arose as a direct result of an individual preference for homogeneity that may have been only slight. In one sense, then, it was this individual preference that caused the neighbourhood character to develop that, in turn, influenced health. However, that health effect would not fit into the usual epidemiological regression equation where risk is a function of individual exposure, in this case the slight preference for homogeneity. We have a true societal-level variable.

This brings us to our third example. Hippocrates drew attention to 'air, water, and places' as characteristics of areas that influence health. We have no difficulty in seeing the quality of air or water as societal-level characteristics. However, so are the quality of schools; so too are the crime rate or the level of unemployment. There is evidence that these societal-level characteristics, part of the social context (Schwartz and Diez-Roux 2001), may influence health not simply because an individual's health suffers as the result of his being unemployed or a victim of crime.

There has been much debate about the validity and measurement of the concept of social capital. We do not propose to settle that debate here. Rather we draw attention to the clear evidence that societal characteristics affect health over and above the characteristics of the individuals who are members of that society. This has been operationalized by examining geographic variation, and there is evidence of interaction between individual-level characteristics and those acting at the societal level (Stafford and Marmot 2003).

Policy and research

The final words of Rose's book are:

> The primary determinants of disease are mainly economic and social, and therefore its remedies must also be economic and social. Medicine and politics cannot and should not be kept apart.

In our view *The Strategy of Preventive Medicine* laid the intellectual foundation for this conclusion. It is a conclusion acknowledged little and acted on less. There are plausible reasons for such neglect. First, those most concerned about the health of populations are in the health sector. The primary concern of the health sector is with treating individuals with disease. Indeed if 'health' spending of governments is examined, it will be found, overwhelmingly, to be on medical care. All governments, and most health professionals, are rightly concerned with treating sick people and relieving suffering. Many in public health have complained that preventing disease and promoting health are seen as minority interests, even when recognized prevention tends to take a particular form. For example, cardiologists have taken over cholesterol. People with raised cholesterol levels become individual patients to be treated with (happily, effective) cholesterol-lowering drugs. This is close to what Rose labelled the high-risk approach.

The population approach leads to a recognition that action needs to be at a societal level. Further, the evidence that we have touched on leads to the conclusion that such intervention needs to be outside the health domain. Important influences on health come from the circumstances in which people live, work, grow, and age. It is precisely because of this recognition that the World Health Organization set up the Commission on Social Determinants of Health (Marmot 2005). As of writing, the Commission has yet to reach its conclusions as to the recommendations it will make on action on the social determinants of health.

There are two issues, and a general principle, that we wish to take up.

Targeted or universal interventions First, should social interventions be targeted at those most in need or should they be universal in nature? This has great resonance with Geoffrey Rose's discussion of high-risk versus population strategy of prevention. The case for targeted interventions appears strong. If poor people have a miserable experience in the education system, then, surely, we should try and improve schools that serve children from impoverished families. If the problem with the poor is that they have insufficient economic resource, then surely the tax and transfer system should be targeted to improve their lot. If crime-ridden neighbourhoods with poor-quality housing and poorly served by amenities damage health, then should we not concentrate on clearing up deprived neighbourhoods?

The case for targeted intervention may appear strong, but there are important caveats. Figure 4 illustrates the literacy levels of offspring according to parents' level of education. There are two striking lessons to be learnt from this figure. First, the relationship between parents' education and literacy of their young adult offspring follows the social gradient. The higher the education of parents, the better their children perform. If we were to target the needy, where would the cut-off point be? The comparison with Sweden shows that the US disadvantage follows the social gradient. At each level of parents' education the Americans do worse than the Swedes. There is, therefore, no clear cut-off. It suggests that performance should

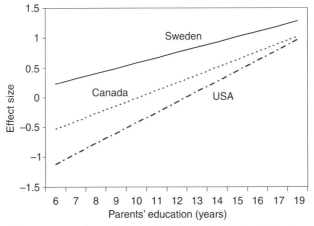

Fig. 4 Literacy scores of people ages 16–25 years by level of education of their parents in the USA, Canada, and Sweden (Willms *et al.* 1999).

be improved across the board in the USA. This leads to the second lesson. Important as parents' education is for the literacy performance of their offspring, it matters where those parents happen to be found. Parents' education may look like destiny in the USA; less so in Sweden. This is consistent with other data that suggest that inter-generational social mobility is actually greater in Scandinavia than it is in the USA.

Whether considering the social gradient that runs across the whole of society, or trying to determine how Swedish levels of social mobility could be transferred to the USA, the implication is that targeting will miss the problem. The appropriate level of intervention may well be the whole of society. Science then rapidly runs into politics. This raises sensitivities to which we shall return at the end of this chapter.

Evidence If remedies are to be economic and social, whether targeted or universal, this brings us to the second issue: what would count as evidence to support proposed policies? There are few within medicine who are other than pleased at the rise of evidence-based medicine. Using simple evaluative methods to focus on which treatments work and weed out those that do not has been a major advance in putting medicine's house in order. To the extent that preventive medicine relies on taking action with individual patients, similar evaluative methods are appropriate. Should an individual be prescribed a statin to lower cholesterol? Only if the evidence shows that the benefit outweighs the risk. The best way of gathering such evidence is a randomized controlled trial.

Parenthetically, we note that a placebo-controlled trial is the most appropriate. So powerful is the effect of patient belief on behaviour and physiological function that most researchers would acknowledge that the placebo effect must be controlled for by design. Even researchers who profess themselves sceptical of the notion that psyche and soma are linked recognize the power of the placebo effect.

Could the same standards of evidence that apply to pharmacological interventions apply to dietary change of individuals? In principle, yes; in practice, with difficulty. Randomized controlled trials of dietary interventions on individuals have been tried with varying success. In large part, the difficulties come from the large numbers needed if disease is the end-point, and the difficulties in 'controlling' behaviour of both the intervention and control groups. The trials of salt and blood pressure that put individuals on low-salt diets and then added sodium to the diets of one group and not the other represent ingenious ways round the problem. People have contemplated such trials with stroke, rather than blood pressure, as an end-point, and shied away from the scale and complexity.

Much has been made of the failure of supplements of antioxidants to prevent cancer or heart disease. Controlled trials have shown that they may be harmful. These trials bring forward good reasons not to prescribe such dietary supplements to prevent cancer or heart disease. They do not represent tests of a dietary hypothesis. The trials of supplements have little to say on whether the type of diet rich in foods of plant origin might be a better diet for prevention of chronic disease than one based on animal foods, low in fibre and rich in fat and refined carbohydrates. A dietary supplement is more akin to a pharmacological intervention, such as post-menopausal oestrogens, and requires rigorous evaluation before it can be prescribed. A dietary change also requires rigorous evaluation, but a trial may not be the most feasible option.

This leads to two further issues to do with evidence. If the proposed intervention is social rather than, say, lifestyle change, the possibilities for evaluation may change. Secondly, if the intervention, following Rose, is to be on the whole population, the possibilities for evaluation may again be limited.

There are examples of social interventions that have been subject to controlled evaluation: the Rand health insurance experiment, the Progressa studies of contingent cash transfer programmes for poor families in Mexico, evaluation of head start programmes in the USA and Sure Start in Britain, and Moving to Opportunity providing improved housing for people in deprived neighbourhoods in the USA. These tend, on the whole, to be programmes targeted at high-risk groups. It is extremely helpful to have such controlled evaluations. The fact that there are but a limited number to cite is perhaps a testament to the difficulty, and expense, of carrying them out.

When we move to interventions on whole populations, the nature of evaluation must change. Would using the taxation system to raise the price of alcohol lead to a drop in alcohol-associated deaths? Probably it would, but it is difficult to envisage a controlled experiment that would prove it. Numerous observational studies show that individuals' alcohol consumption is sensitive to price—hardly a surprise as this is a foundation of economics. Different observational studies show that population consumption of alcohol follows, inversely, the real price of alcohol. Still more observational studies show that alcohol-associated harm appears to be correlated with mean consumption levels in the population. Putting it together, there is a reasonable judgement that one way of reducing alcohol-associated harm in the population is to raise the real price of alcohol (Academy of Medical Sciences 2004). This is evidence-based policy formulation but it is not the same type of evidence that forms the gold standard for evaluating pharmacological interventions.

If, to take the example cited earlier, the judgement is that social capital is importantly related to health of communities, it may be possible to formulate evidence-based policy recommendations on actions that could be taken to improve social capital. It is unlikely that such evidence will include randomized controlled evaluations.

We are familiar with this in other areas of policy making. Is an independent central bank good or bad for the economy? Does Keynesian-style economic intervention provide better solutions to economic cycles than strict control of the money supply? Do comprehensive schools lead to greater social cohesion than selective schools? Would regulation or economic instruments, such as trading permits, be a better way to deal with climate change? These are all crucial questions that affect the lives of the public (and perhaps even their health) that in the main have to be settled without recourse to randomized controlled trials.

Population action

As Rose said, echoing Virchow, medicine and politics cannot and should not be kept apart. As scientists, we are concerned with providing the evidence for interventions, but the acceptability of interventions touches on fundamental issues. We can illustrate with two examples that have been touched on above: alcohol and social inequalities in health.

Rose's high-risk versus population approach applies well to alcohol. A high-risk approach would suggest that the appropriate target for intervention should be heavy drinkers. A population approach recognizes that overall mean consumption predicts alcohol-associated harm and therefore the intervention should be on the whole population through mechanisms such as higher prices and restricted availability. In the UK, for example, as the real price of alcohol has plummeted over the last 30 years, and availability become easier, mean alcohol consumption of the population has doubled, and harm, such as cirrhosis mortality, has increased correspondingly.

A government that is terrified of being labelled an agent of the 'nanny state' would opt for the first: targeting heavy or nuisance drinkers. The alcohol industry, likewise, would sign up to the first but not the second: by all means get rid of heavy drinkers but do not reduce mean alcohol consumption. The high-risk approach fits well with a strategy that calls for targeting the problem where it occurs. It also has the advantage that it deals with the perceived fundamental flaw of the population approach to control of alcohol consumption. Why should individual moderate drinkers, who are unlikely to be harmed by their drinking, have to endure methods such as higher prices or restricted availability?

These are huge and important political/philosophical questions. We have all heard the refrains. I am a safe driver why should there be a law requiring me to wear a seat belt? If I want fluoride I'll take it; it does not need to be in the water supply. Why should we cyclists stop at red lights if we cause no harm to others? If I want to use morphine or cocaine surely that's my business. There are clearly two parts of the argument: what works and what is politically acceptable. If a group is philosophically opposed to population interventions they may as well know if interventions aimed at high-risk heavy drinkers are ineffective. At least they know they are pushing a side of the argument that would not solve the problem. Conversely if the evidence supported a population intervention but the proposed societal change was unacceptable, it is well to have public deliberation over such issues.

What is surely unacceptable is to have population interventions without public deliberation. These cannot be reduced to issues of the political right versus the political left. Genetically modified foods are a good example. The evidence base for or against widespread introduction into the food supply may be inadequate, but that does not justify introduction of these foods without adequate public deliberation as to their acceptability.

Our other example comes from interventions to reduce inequalities in health. Evidence such as that presented in Fig. 4 (p. 22) for literacy shows that the health inequality problem does not reduce to poor health for the poor and good health for everyone else. Yet many would see the problem of poor health for the poor as something requiring action but be quite resistant to changes for the whole population. They would be comfortable with targeted action: more money for schools in deprived areas, opening of new medical facilities in such areas, programmes to improve access, and support for single mothers in poverty. They would find an approach to improving the whole of society, such as a Scandinavian-type welfare regime, unacceptable politically whatever the evidence for its effect on reducing inequalities in health of the population.

Conclusions

While population-based interventions, aimed at shifting the whole population distribution by some mass strategy to alter widespread exposures, are the ones with much greater potential impact on the total numbers of individual cases, compared with individual interventions, causal certainty is much less for population exposures compared with individual exposures. As Schwartz and Diez-Roux (2001) have pointed out, where epidemiology may diverge from more reductionist approaches, or where epidemiologists may even disagree amongst themselves, is in the criteria used to assess causal models. Usually, the greatest emphasis is placed on the certainty and universality of the association; and, of course, the simpler and more proximal the model, the greater the certainty. However, if the aim is to improve human health, causal priority is not based on the certainty of the causal attribution but on the efficiency with which the removal of the cause could potentially reduce the incidence, or overall burden, of disease. The causes about which aetiological significances are most certain are the proximal ones, but the closer in the causal chain the less the opportunity for prevention. The dilemma is that the further back in the causal chain, the greater the prevention opportunities but also the lower the certainty about causes.

Rose recognized the potential difficulties of both the individual and population approaches to prevention summarized in Table 5. To have a substantial impact on the population, a mass strategy is required which aims at shifting the population mean. However, this approach raises several dilemmas. Evidence to support mass strategies is very limited. It is much more difficult to identify the complex determinants of population distributions with any certainty and to conduct randomized trials in populations. There is lack of understanding of the nature of the risk relationship: shifting the distribution may have benefits for one end but disbenefits for the other end of the distribution. The complexity of population changes and unforeseen outcomes means that small changes may have large benefits but also potentially unforeseen disbenefits. Thus at one extreme, it has been stated that public health strategies require something approaching certainty, and altering population risk is an unreal aspiration. There is often a lack of incentive for individuals, as exemplified by the vaccination example. Large numbers of people are exposed and, when disease is prevented, no specific individuals can be identified who have benefited but people who are harmed by side effects are easily identified. Additionally, the need to target resources to those who would benefit most is pressing.

A corollary to the mass strategy in prevention which aims to change the prevalence of disease is that we need to consider what the likely impact on the prevalence of extremes may be in any policies that are

Table 5 Strategies of prevention

Individual based	Population based	
Identify individuals at high risk: screening	Identify important risk factors for the community (prevalence)	
Intervene only in individuals at high risk	Policy to reduce risk factor irrespective of individual risk	
Risk–benefit balance individually ssessed	Risk–benefit balance for whole community	
	Individual intervention	**Population intervention**
Individuals identified	Yes	No
Potential benefits for individual	Large	Small
Potential benefits for population	Small	Large
Understanding of effects	Good	Poor

likely to influence population norms. As the examples from gambling and alcohol use suggest, policies that affect population norms also influence the prevalence of problem drinkers or problem gamblers, respectively, and it is not difficult to speculate on the many other areas in which this might apply, for example changing laws on drug use, or average speed limits on roads.

Rose acknowledged the imperfect evidence base and complexity of society, the unlikelihood of a universal right answer; and hence the need for constant assessment of impact. Rose suggests that since we can never be totally certain of anything, action depends on the consequences of making the wrong decision either way; and should proceed alongside continuing assessment and evaluation of the evidence. The adequacy or otherwise of scientific evidence should be judged in the context of the particular use to which it is to be put.

Even in the era of gene discovery and individualized medicine, the wide and disparate range of examples in which the single population model can be shown to apply reaffirm Rose's statement that:

The essential determinants of the health of society are thus to be found in its mass characteristics: the deviant minority can only be understood when seen in its societal context and effective prevention requires changes which involve the population as a whole.

In his original preface, he said 'The purpose of this book is … to explore … the often disturbing implications for policy, research, and ethics of the population-wide approach to the prevention of common medical and behavioural disorders.' Indeed, 'The health of society is integral, and the supposedly "normal" majority needs to accept responsibility for its deviant minority—however loth it may be to do so'.

References

Academy of Medical Sciences (2004). *Calling time: the nation's drinking as a major health issue*. London: Academy of Medical Sciences.

Anderson, J., Huppert, F., and Rose, G. (1993). Normality, deviance and minor psychiatric morbidity in the community. A population-based approach to General Health Questionnaire data in the Health and Lifestyle Survey. *Psychol. Med.* **23**, 475–485.

Batchelor, P. and Sheiham, A. (2002). The limitations of a 'high-risk' approach for the prevention of dental caries. *Community Dent. Oral Epidemiol.* **30**, 302–312.

De Backer, G., Ambrosioni, E., Borch-Johnsen, K., Brotons, C., Cifkova, R., Dallongeville, J., *et al.* (2003). European guidelines on cardiovascular disease prevention in clinical practice: third joint task force of European and other societies on cardiovascular disease prevention in clinical practice (constituted by representatives of eight societies and by invited experts). *Eur. J. Cardiovasc. Prev. Rehabil.* **10**, S1–S10.

Emberson, J., Whincup, P., Morris, R., Walker, M., and Ebrahim, S. (2004). Evaluating the impact of population and high-risk strategies for the primary prevention of cardiovascular disease. *Eur. Heart J.* **25**, 484–491.

Fechtner, R.D. and Khouri, A.S. (2007). Evolving global risk assessment of ocular hypertension to glaucoma. *Curr. Opin. Ophthalmol.* **18**, 104–109.

Ford, E., Ajani, U., Croft, J., Cirtchley, J., Labarthe, D., Kottke, T., *et al.* (2007). Explaining the decrease in US deaths from coronary heart disease, 1980–2000. *N. Engl. J. Med.* **356**, 2388–2398.

Frayling, T.M., Timpson, N.J., Weedon, M.N., Zeggini, E., Freathy, R.M., Lindgren, C.M., *et al.* (2007). A common variant in the FTO gene is associated with body mass index and predisposes to childhood and adult obesity. *Science* **316**, 889–894.

Grun, L. and McKeigue, P. (2000). Prevalence of excessive gambling before and after introduction of a national lottery in the United Kingdom: another example of the single distribution theory. *Addiction* **95**, 959–966.

Kanis, J.A., Oden, A., Johnell, O., Johansson, H., De Laet, C., Brown, J., *et al.* (2007). The use of clinical risk factors enhances the performance of BMD in the prediction of hip and osteoporotic fractures in men and women. *Osteoporos. Int.* **18**, 1033–1046.

Khaw, K.T., Wareham, N., Bingham, S., Luben, R., Welch, A., and Day, N. (2004*a*). Association of hemoglobin A1c with cardiovascular disease and mortality in adults: the European prospective investigation into cancer in Norfolk. *Ann. Intern. Med.* **141**, 413–420.

Khaw, K.T., Reeve, J., Luben, R., Bingham, S., Welch, A., Wareham, N., *et al.* (2004*b*). Prediction of total and hip fracture risk in men and women by quantitative ultrasound of the calcaneus: EPIC-Norfolk prospective population study. *Lancet* **363**, 197–202.

Leske, M.C., Wu, S.Y., Nemesure, B., and Hennis, A. (2002). Incident open-angle glaucoma and blood pressure. *Arch. Ophthalmol.* **120**, 954–959.

Marmot, M. (2005). Social determinants of health inequalities. *Lancet* **365**, 1099–1104.

Mokdad, A.H., Serdula, M.K., Dietz, W.H., Bowman, B.A., Marks, J.S., and Koplan, J.P. (1999). The spread of the obesity epidemic in the United States, 1991–1998. *JAMA* **282**, 1519–1522.

Mullis, I., Martin, M., Gonzalez, E., and Chrostowski, S. (2004). *Findings from IEA's Trends in International Mathematics and Science Study at the fourth and eighth grades.* Chestnut Hill, MA: TIMSS & PIRLS International Study Center, Boston College.

Schelling, T. (1978). *Micromotives and macrobehaviour.* New York: Norton.

Schwartz S, Diez-Roux AV. (2001). Commentary: causes of incidence and causes of cases–a Durkheimian perspective on Rose. *Int. J. Epidemiol.* **30**, 435–439.

Stafford, M. and Marmot, M. (2003). Neighbourhood deprivation and health: does it affect us all equally? *Int. J. Epidemiol.* **32**, 357–366.

Willms, J.D. (1999). Inequalities in literacy skills among youth in Canada and the United States (International Adjult Literacy Survey no 6). Ottawa: Human Resources Development Canada and National Literacy Secretariat.

The Strategy of Preventive Medicine

Geoffrey Rose

Chapter 1

The objectives of preventive medicine

The scope for prevention

Few diseases are the inescapable lot of humanity, for a problem that is common in one place will usually prove to be rare somewhere else. Cervical cancer is twenty times commoner in Colombia than in Israel, 10 per cent of Indian children die before their first birthday whereas in Western countries 99 per cent of babes survive, and according to UK census figures 3.1 per cent of adults in Wales report that they are permanently sick, compared with only 1.2 per cent of residents in southeast England. There is no known biological reason why every population should not be as healthy as the best.

Virchow, the great German pathologist of the last century, wrote:

Epidemics appear, and often disappear without traces, when a new culture period has started; thus with leprosy, and the English sweat. The history of epidemics is therefore the history of disturbances of human culture (Virchow, in Ackerknecht 1970).

Soon after he wrote this, coronary heart disease emerged from obscurity to become the commonest cause of death in Western countries; now it is on the wane. In countries with a newly expanding economy, such as Hong Kong, the old historical pattern of sickness (high infant mortality, and adult deaths mostly due to infections) is now giving way to the problems of heart attack and duodenal ulcer.

The scale and pattern of disease reflect the way that people live and their social, economic, and environmental circumstances, and all of these can change quickly. This implies that most diseases are, in theory, preventable, but it leaves us with some anxious questions. Can we control our history, or must we only analyse and observe it?

Is there an ideal way of life which will minimize every threat to health? Can we hope simultaneously to avoid on the one hand the ills of poverty and the simple life, and on the other hand the ills of affluence and industrialization?

Why seek to prevent?

'Take no thought for the morrow … sufficient unto the day is the evil thereof' (Matthew, Chapter 6, Verse 34). This injunction touches a deeply held human feeling that it may be better to live a day at a time rather than to be anxious about distant problems which may never materialize. Doctors often act as though their professional responsibility does not go beyond the sick and the nearly sick (those at imminent risk), and politicians, who influence health more than the doctors, are rarely troubled by thoughts for the distant future.

Concern for future health is a luxury item—all the efforts of the poor and the unemployed are needed to cope with more pressing immediate problems. Rising prosperity, however, liberates people from some of these immediate practical demands, so that nowadays we witness a rising interest in health, healthy living, and a healthy environment. This raises a conflict between on the one hand prudence, which encourages precautions now from which we may later reap benefits, and on the other hand a danger of neurotic anxiety.

The economic argument

The case for preventive medicine is often argued on economic grounds. Ill health impairs earning capacity, and the costs of medical care are high and continually escalating; prevention, it is said, will be a money-saver. On closer scrutiny this argument may prove misleading or even false, for several reasons. In the first place, success often means the postponement of a problem rather than its ultimate prevention. For example, the avoidance of cigarettes will greatly reduce the risks at each age of suffering a heart attack, but as a result non-smokers live longer and so more of them are exposed to the particularly high risk of heart attack in old age. The paradoxical result is that, even though smoking indeed causes heart attacks, non-smokers are more likely than smokers to die (eventually) of such an attack (Rose and Shipley 1990). Avoidance of smoking is excellent preventive advice, offering the prospect of a healthier and longer life, but surprisingly it may, as an isolated measure, actually increase the number of heart attacks. The corresponding costs are then postponed rather than avoided.

Success in reducing the overall incidence rate of a common disease ought in theory to reduce the health service costs, since there are fewer cases to be treated. In practice this hope tends to be frustrated by the continually rising costs of investigating and treating each patient, and by the ingenuity of health service staff. Thus the massive decline in dental caries has not led to any corresponding fall in the number of dentists or their level of activity; nor has the widespread decline in the incidence of coronary heart disease led to any fall in the numbers of cardiologists and cardiac surgeons. In fact, the costs of investigation and care have been inversely related to the changes in incidence! A dynamic relationship between medical care costs and epidemiologically established needs has proved hard to establish.

Despite these negative observations it would be wrong to overlook other examples where a decline in the incidence of a disease (tuberculosis, for instance) has indeed brought large savings. Even here, however, the argument of overall economic advantage may be fallacious, for every death avoided, whether by prevention or treatment, means one extra old person, and old people are economically unproductive whilst at the same time costly, both medically and in their needs for social support.

My economist friends tell me that the death of a newborn babe is of small economic interest to society, for the infant has cost little to produce and in money terms will cost little to replace. The death of young adults, by contrast, is a grievous economic loss: they have been expensive to rear and educate, and their death means a loss of many productive years. Thus an investment in the prevention of road traffic accidents, which particularly involve young adults, would indeed be economically advantageous, as too would any success in preventing AIDS. Somewhere around age 50, so the economists say, is the balance point, where the benefits of a few more productive years are more or less equivalent to the added costs of surviving into old age. Beyond that age the economic argument for prevention undergoes progressive collapse, for alas the cheapest patient is a dead patient!

So far as health service costs are concerned the economic argument for prevention may often fail to meet expectations except where, as has been the case with tuberculosis, the occurrence of the disease so diminishes that a whole sector of services can be closed down. If the argument is widened to include the total economic balance-sheet for society, then it seems that the prevention of deaths is only likely to involve net economic advantage if it applies to children or young adults, and beyond the age of about 50 the economic outcome is increasingly negative as applied to preventive measures which extend survival. However, at every age before retirement there is an economic gain from any preventive policy which can reduce disability or improve working capacity, and after retirement there are economic savings from anything which enhances independence and reduces the need for medical and social supports.

The humanitarian argument

It is better to be healthy than ill or dead. That is the beginning and the end of the only real argument for preventive medicine. It is sufficient.

Priorities: a matter of choice

The knowledge that we already possess is sufficient, if put into practice, to achieve great health gains for all and to reduce our scandalous international and national inequalities in health. What impedes its translation into action? Some of the reasons are wholly deplorable, including widespread ignorance and lack of understanding of the issues and possibilities, and the deliberate opposition of powerful vested interests. Such obstacles to better health need to be exposed and opposed.

Other reasons, however, are not matters for assertion but for debate and choice. The achievement of better health implies many kinds of costs which must be paid if we want good preventive medical services, a healthier environment, and better conditions of work, travel, and housing. If people wish it to be so, these ends can be achieved, but only if they are willing to transfer resources from other uses, peaceful or military. Similarly, changes to a healthier life-style imply personal costs, which individuals must balance against their valuation of health. If I were to put an unlimited valuation on my health, I should probably adopt a Japanese diet, as the Japanese are the longest-lived people in the world. That would be possible, but as I do not live in Japan, the cost to my domestic and social life would be high, and I do not value health as much as that! Similarly the smoker has to decide whether the health and other benefits of stopping are worth the loss of a pleasure and the difficulties of giving up.

The task of preventive medicine is not to tell people what they should do. That is a matter for societies and their individual members to decide. The purpose of this book is to analyse the options, so that such important choices can be based on a clearer understanding of the issues.

Chapter 2

What needs to be prevented?

Those who seek to remedy the world's ills like to see situations in clear and dichotomous terms: doctors categorize people as sick or healthy, social reformers and politicians focus their concerns on definable minorities and discrete problem areas, moralists identify choices as black or white, evangelists see a world made up of the converted and the heathen, and so on. Any alternative creates indecision and uncertainty.

Sick individuals

Concern for sick individuals has led to an attractively simple approach to preventive medicine. We wish to reduce the number of sick individuals, who form a clearly definable minority; by implication the majority of the population is normal and should therefore be left in peace. This approach rests on the traditional principle of medical diagnosis which assumes that, with respect to each disease, the world falls into just two classes, namely those who have it and those who do not. Thus if a patient comes to clinic complaining of pain in the belly, the doctor must consider a series of possible diagnoses (peptic ulcer, gastric cancer, gallstones, and so on), and for each there must be a simple judgement, 'yes' or 'no', implying that each condition is either present or absent. This is the diagnostic process.

This simple model of disease has always dominated medical thinking. It went virtually unquestioned until 1954, when George Pickering advanced the revolutionary proposal that the idea of a sharp distinction between health and disease is a medical artefact for which nature, if consulted, provides no support (Hamilton *et al.* 1954). I was his medical registrar at the time, and I well remember the widespread bafflement which greeted this famous professor of medicine when he asserted that hypertension, in which he was the world expert, did not

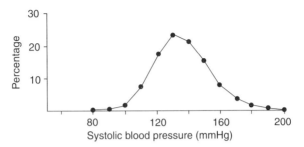

Fig. 2.1 Disease and its risk factors are quantitative not categorical phenomena: the distribution of systolic blood pressure in a population of middle-aged men.

exist as a distinguishable entity. Devious but determined attempts were made to demonstrate overt or hidden bimodality in the blood pressure distribution, and for many months this argument dominated the correspondence columns of *The Lancet*. Finally Pickering won his point, for it had to be admitted that blood pressure does indeed come in all degrees, with 'low' merging imperceptibly into 'high' (Fig. 2.1).

This fact could not be gainsaid, but neither the fact nor Pickering's powerful advocacy was able to alter medicine's underlying commitment to the belief that a disease must be either present or absent. Pickering later wrote

Essential hypertension is a type of disease not hitherto recognized in medicine in which the defect is quantitative not qualitative. It is difficult for doctors to understand because it is a departure from the ordinary process of binary thought to which they are brought up. Medicine in its present state can count up to two but not beyond. (Pickering 1968)

Thus Pickering may have won the battle but he lost the war. Indeed, he never realized that this penetrating insight into the nature of hypertension has far-reaching implications in many other health and social fields. The notions presented in this book spring directly from his original concept, but they generalize it to other areas and explore its relevance to preventive policy.

A continuum of disease severity

The demand for clear definitions has dominated epidemiological research. John Snow was only able to demonstrate that cholera is spread by polluted water supplies because he could locate and count the cases of cholera and then calculate attack rates according to the source of water supply. Subsequently most health statistics and most epidemiological research have continued to be based on the counting of cases, which in turn rests on the assumption that disease can be clearly defined and separated from normality.

Paradoxically, it is epidemiological research which has now repeatedly demonstrated that in fact disease is nearly always a quantitative rather than a categorical or qualitative phenomenon, and hence it has no natural definitions. What Pickering first showed to be true of hypertension is now seen to be the norm rather than the exception. Infectious diseases in the population also come in all sizes, from obvious 'clinical' cases down to symptomless infections that are only revealed by special laboratory tests. The clinical illness recognized as cancer is the infrequent end-stage of a series of common changes, beginning with minor cellular abnormalities (metaplasia) and ranging through more definitely premalignant change (dysplasia), localized (*in situ*) malignancy, and locally invasive disease. Interruption of cerebral blood flow can lead to a whole spectrum of consequences ranging from none at all, or symptoms too mild to come to any medical attention, through a 'transient ischaemic attack' (defined, quite arbitrarily, as a stroke that recovers with 24 hours), to a stroke with persistent disability or a dramatic and rapidly fatal illness. Even pregnancy is not defined by nature, but rather it develops in a series of steps from the merely potential (a sperm swimming towards an ovum), through the stages of fertilized ovum, implantation in the uterus (apparently the legal definition), a biochemically detectable pregnancy, a clinically evident pregnancy, a recognizably human fetus, a viable fetus, and finally a live baby. The answer to 'When does a new life begin?' is thus an arbitrary issue, not a natural fact. Even the distinction between human and subhuman receives little support from nature.

Senile dementia is widely regarded as a distinct entity, and much research effort goes into looking for 'the causes of Alzheimer's disease', yet epidemiological study of cognitive function in an elderly population finds that 'normality' merges imperceptibly into 'dementia', suggesting that we should move away from asking 'Has he got it?' towards 'How much of it has he got, and why?' (Brayne and Calloway 1988).

In each of these instances nature presents us with a process or continuum and not a dichotomy. Exceptions are few and far between, being largely confined to a handful of congenital disorders determined by a single dominant gene with high penetrance. For example, there can be no argument about recognizing an achondroplastic dwarf, for no one can have 'a touch of dwarfism': the condition is either present or absent. Far more often, however, even when a disorder has a simple genetic basis its expression is greatly modified by other associated factors; thus among those with the genotype for Wilson's disease some die early of liver failure whilst others have a biochemical abnormality of copper excretion but remain in seemingly good health. Nearly all diseases, whether genetic or acquired, come in all sizes.

Case definitions

The practical necessity for case definitions is nevertheless obvious and has always been recognized. The decision to ban lepers from human society presupposed a confident ability to know who was or was not a leper: the possibility of mistakes in either direction was not to be contemplated, and to recognize 'a touch of leprosy' would have been very confusing. When a woman attends an antenatal clinic there can be no shilly-shallying about whether her blood pressure is high: if it is, then she must be admitted to hospital, but if not, she can go home. In this way most clinical decisions are dichotomous: the patient is either admitted or allowed home, a drug is given in full dose or not at all, and an operation is or is not performed. A clear-cut decision presupposes a clear-cut diagnosis.

This creates an illogical situation. Disease truly forms a continuum of severity, but its management requires a system of unambiguous labels. The big mistake has been, not the use of dichotomous diagnostics, but to consider that process as being a description of the natural order rather than merely an operational convenience. Management policy requires 'yes/no' decisions such as investigate or not investigate, admit or send home, treat or not treat. This decision-taking underlies the process we choose to call 'diagnosis', but what that really means is that we are diagnosing 'a case for treatment' and not a disease entity. Although the psychiatrist picks out certain individuals who are labelled as 'cases of depression', what is really meant is 'cases for anti-depressive treatment', for depression itself occurs in all grades of severity and most never come to the psychiatrist's attention.

If diseases come in all grades of severity then this widens the task of preventive medicine. It is an inappropriate limitation, reflecting the particular outlook of doctors, to suppose that we only need to reduce the number of people requiring medical care. To improve the nation's health statistics for consultations, hospital admissions, and mortality is indeed an important measure of preventive success, but it is not sufficient for it fails to consider that much of the population's burden of ill health derives from a mass of less obvious troubles which doctors do not see. For example, in our studies of angina we found that only about a quarter of all the sufferers had ever been diagnosed. There is a vast submerged burden of ill health. This is not necessarily treatable, but we ought to seek means for its prevention.

Doctors tend to give the highest priority to the prevention of death and acute illness, whereas members of the public may attach more importance to how they feel and to impairments of daily living. The two outlooks imply different views of ill health. Table 2.1 contrasts, for various countries, the subjective perception of health status with an objective medical measure. It is impossible to say that either is a more valid description of ill health than the other, because they measure different things.

Preventive medicine should be concerned with the whole spectrum of disease and ill health, both because all levels are important to the people concerned and because the mild can be the father of the severe. The visible tip of the iceberg of disease can be neither understood nor properly controlled if it is thought to constitute the entire problem.

A continuum of risk

Figure 2.2 shows the relation between blood pressure and the risk of stroke or heart attack. Current policy is to recommend that all adults should have their blood pressure measured, with drug treatment then

Table 2.1 Proportion of people in various countries who regard their health as 'very good', compared with the corresponding figures for life expectancy

Country	Percentage reporting 'health very good'	Life expectancy (years)
Ireland	48	71.6
USA	40	71.6
UK	39	72.4
Sweden	38	74.2
Australia	36	73.2
France	19	72.0
Italy	15	72.7
Japan	9	75.9
USSR	3	65.1

Source: International Gallup Polls; World Health Organization 1989, 1990

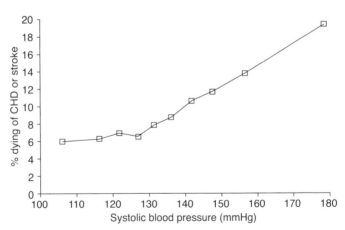

Fig. 2.2 Relation between systolic blood pressure in middle-aged men and the risk (age-adjusted) of suffering fatal coronary heart disease (CHD) or stroke in the next 18 years (Whitehall Study).

being considered if the diastolic value exceeds about 100 mmHg. This policy has prevented a great many strokes, but it has also done harm by encouraging the belief that those who do not qualify for the high-risk group, because they are 'normal', have no cause for concern. The figure shows this belief to be false: just as Pickering demonstrated a continuum of blood pressure, so there is also a continuum of associated risk which increases progressively over the whole observed range.

The prevention paradox

It is a common irony of preventive medicine that many people must take precautions in order to prevent illness in only a few. Even 50 years ago, when diphtheria was rampant, several hundred children had to be immunized in order to prevent one death—all because no one could say which child was destined for calamity. Assuming that the wearing of a car seat belt halves the risk of death to the driver, the odds that a particular individual will ever benefit are of the order of several hundred to one against: happily, few of us were going to be killed on the roads anyway. This common phenomenon has been expressed as the 'prevention paradox' (Rose 1981): *a preventive measure that brings large benefits to the community offers little to each participating individual.*

This distressing paradox implies that a response to honest health education is unlikely to be motivated powerfully by the prospect of better health. Whether or not a middle-aged smoker chooses to give up his cigarettes may affect his chances of being alive in 20 years time by less than 10 per cent (Rose and Colwell 1992). Similarly, a decision to lose some excess weight, to take regular exercise, or to use soft margarine in lieu of butter—each a prudent step to take—will make only a tiny difference to a particular person's health prospects, at least in the next few years. People are generally motivated only by the prospect of a benefit which is visible, early, and likely. Health benefits rarely meet these criteria; they may be real, but they are likely to be delayed and to come to only a few of those who seek them.

Happily this does not mean that health education has no chance, but only that its acceptance depends on attractions other than a distant hope of better health. The anti-smoking effort has achieved a radical change in public attitudes, for a habit which a few years ago was considered normal is now widely disapproved of, even by smokers. The motivation for this change has been more social and psychological than medical, because a person who gives up cigarettes is immediately rewarded by enhanced self-esteem and social approval. Thus unhealthy behaviour involves a usually small and remote risk of damage to health but also an immediately perceptible damage to self-respect.

Mass measures and individual measures

Some preventive measures can, by their very nature, only be implemented on a mass scale. This applies, for example, to public services such as fluoridation of water supply and to environmental measures such as legislative control of air pollution, and health education by the mass media is necessarily indiscriminate. In contrast, when preventive measures are applied at the individual level (which would include the earlier examples of immunization and car seat belts) it is inefficient to offer them to everyone when only a minority will reap a benefit.

The search for more efficient preventive policies leads to the *high-risk strategy*, in which efforts are focused on those individuals who are judged mostly likely to develop disease. This avoids the wastefulness of the mass approach, with its need to interfere with people most of whom neither ask for help nor will benefit from it.

This high-risk strategy of prevention implies segregation of a minority with special problems from a majority who are regarded as normal and not needing attention. Whether or not this is reasonable depends on the extent to which a particular risk is indeed confined to an identifiable minority, but our ability to discriminate in this way may be inadequate. Concern for the welfare of individuals may be good for these particular people, but concern for the health of the public as a whole points us in a different direction. We need to consider the implications of a situation in which a small risk involves a large number of people, who in the high-risk strategy would be categorized as normal. The result for the population may be a large number of cases, even though no one was at a conspicuous risk. A *population strategy* of prevention is necessary wherever risk is widely diffused through the whole population (Rose 1985).

A unified approach to prevention

The clinical or high-risk approach to prevention has tended to concentrate attention on the conspicuous segment of disease and risk, seeking to understand and control it as though it were the whole of the problem and failing to recognize its integral links with the state of the population in general. Conversely, those taking the public health or environmentalist approach have often been suspicious of medicalization and doctors, and this has isolated them from mainstream medicine, from first-hand experience of illness and disease, and from relevant biological insights.

The succeeding chapters will explore the principles and ramifications of the high-risk and population strategies of prevention, and their respective strengths and limitations. Finally, the conclusion will be that preventive medicine must embrace both, but, of the two, power resides with the population strategy.

Chapter 3

The relation of risk to exposure

The dose–effect relationship

The shape of the dose–effect curve is critical for the planning of control policy. Figure 3.1 illustrates schematically four possibilities, with some examples. Each of the four carries quite different policy implications.

In Fig. 3.1(a) exposure is without adverse effects until it reaches a certain high level, beyond which the risk increases rapidly. This applies, for example, to intraocular pressure, which can vary over a wide range ('the normal range') without any problems, but when it exceeds the critical level there is a rapid rise in the incidence of glaucoma (one of the commonest causes of preventable blindness). It also applies to anaemia and its associated symptoms, for there is no evident disadvantage to being mildly anaemic and hence there may be no benefit if treatment is given in order to raise a haemoglobin level of, say, 10 g/dl up to the 'normal' level of 14.8 g/dl (Elwood 1973). It is generally supposed, though on inadequate evidence, that a curve of this type also describes the relationship between the level of blood alcohol and the risk of involvement in a road traffic accident, and this is the basis for punishing drivers whose levels exceed the 'legal' limit whilst condoning lower levels. (Some countries, such as Norway, punish any driver found to have detectable alcohol in the blood, perhaps with the aim of deterrence rather than from any different view on the dose–effect curve.)

Figure 3.1(b) shows a linear dose–effect relationship over the whole range of exposure. Any level has to be regarded as hazardous, with the excess of adverse effects being in simple proportion to the dose received. This is exemplified by the case of cigarette smoking and lung cancer, where the risk of disease relative to that for a non-smoker is

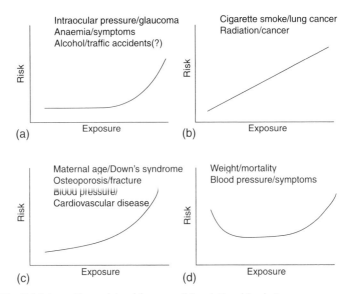

Fig. 3.1 Schematic models of four possible relationships between exposure to a cause and the associated risk of disease.

about the same as the number of cigarettes smoked daily, and even the very small dose received through 'passive' smoking carries a small but real increase in cancer incidence (to the great alarm of the manufacturers). Removal of the hazard would require a total end to exposure.

A threshold-free linear relationship is also accepted as the theoretical basis for policy on radiation exposure: it is supposed that there is no such thing as a safe dose, with the risk of induced cancers being thought to rise progressively over the whole range. Again, this implies that an ideal policy would totally eliminate all avoidable exposure. The price, however, is too great, since it would mean an end to medical X-rays, as well as to the nuclear industry. This introduces the extremely tricky notion of determining the level of 'acceptable risk'.

There is an accelerating proliferation of regulations which set standards for maximum permitted exposures–for the workplace in industry, for food additives or contaminants, for impurities in the environment or the water supply, for residual monomers in plastics, and for many other hazards. It is important to be clear whether it is supposed that the standard corresponds to a threshold, below which exposure carries no risk (Fig. 3.1(a)), or whether the true relationship has no such threshold (Fig. 3.1(b)), in which case it should be acknowledged openly that a compromise has had to be reached between concern for health and the economic and social costs. The public is often led to believe that exposure below the set limit is safe, whereas in reality there is a risk but the standards authority has decided that it is 'acceptable'. Regrettably, we often do not know which of the models shown in Fig. 3.1(a) or 3.1(b) applies, and so the setting of an 'acceptable' level of exposure again involves a compromise, which ought to be acknowledged. A possible risk is still a risk.

A straight-line relationship such as that shown in Fig. 3.1(b) is usually an oversimplification, reflecting inadequate data. Some sort of curved relationship, such as that shown in Fig. 3.1(c), is more likely, but it needs a lot of data to demonstrate it. There are many examples of such a relationship. The incidence of Down's syndrome increases over the whole range of maternal age, but the slope is shallow below about 30 years. Screening policy often takes this as a critical level; this seems reasonable, because risk becomes high at older ages but is very low, though not absent, for the younger mothers.

The alarming increase in fractures of the neck of the femur in old people has focused our interest on the predisposing role of osteoporosis. The relationship seems to be approximately exponential: the most solid bones are the least likely to fracture, but it is only with the more severe degrees of osteoporosis that the individual's excess risk becomes worrying. A similar relationship exists between either blood pressure or blood cholesterol and the risk of heart attack or stroke.

There is here a dual implication for preventive strategy. High-risk individuals exist and should if possible be helped, but most people also face a small and potentially avoidable problem, and so their level of exposure should be reduced if possible.

Figure 3.1(d) sets out a more complex situation, yet one which fits in readily with the popular lay notion that 'moderation is good, extremism is bad'. It portrays a wide central band within which there is no cause for concern, but with an increasing risk among the deviants at either extreme. For example, there is no such thing as an 'ideal weight' for an adult, but rather a range of satisfactory weights;

mortality rates are higher not only among the obese but also (though to a lesser extent) among those who are conspicuously thin. The same is approximately true of the relation of birth weight to perinatal mortality, for small babies fare badly but so also do very large babies (though to a lesser extent) and birth weight then identifies two different high risk groups. A policy which increased the average birth weight by a shift in the whole distribution would in theory bring some losses as well as gains.

British physicians have long pooh-poohed the belief of their French colleagues that low blood pressure can make people feel tired and weak. Recent evidence gives some support to the French view: the association at least exists, though causality is unproven (Wessely *et al.* 1990). Any health burden from low blood pressure is small in comparison with the strokes and heart attacks caused by high blood pressure, but it ought at least to be borne in mind when debating a policy which aims at a general reduction of blood pressure levels in the population. Might such a policy increase the number of tired people, and if so, by how much?

The limitations of research

Much of the best research is undertaken out of intellectual curiosity, but although the advancement of learning is indeed an excellent thing in itself and the main stimulus to excellence, one sometimes wishes for better communications between academia and the world of decisions and action. In particular there should be more support for applied epidemiology ('public health epidemiology').

The first questions which a science research grants committee usually asks of an application are 'Is the hypothesis clearly stated?' and 'Will the study be able to show if the hypothesis is false?'. Results are expected to be either positive ('statistically significant') or negative, indicating that a particular exposure is or is not associated with disease, or a particular intervention is or is not effective. The actual size of effects is usually estimated only in terms of the relative risk (for aetiology) or proportionate benefit (for an intervention).

All this is far removed from the world of health policy. Relative risk is not what decision-taking requires, for doubling a trivial risk is still trivial but doubling a common risk is alarming. 'Relative risk' is only for researchers; decisions call for absolute measures. The same applies to describing the effects of an intervention: there is small gain from a 10 per cent reduction in a rare risk, whereas a similar reduction for a common disease would be a major advance. What we need to know in order to determine policy is not simply 'Is there an effect?' (answer 'yes' or 'no'), but rather 'How big is the effect?'.

Unfortunately, in order to estimate magnitude with any useful degree of precision often requires a very large study. In our survey of mortality among employees of the UK Atomic Energy Authority (Beral *et al.* 1985) we set out to measure the effects of low-dose radiation by following the mortality outcome among 39 546 workers over an average period of 16 years. Despite the large size of this study the statistical confidence limits on the results were wide, so that we could not say whether the International Commission on Radiological Protection had set a standard which on the one hand was too high, or on the other hand might have been 15-fold too low.

This shows the difficulty of estimating even the overall strength of an effect, and this in a group with relatively high exposure. One can imagine then the mind-boggling demands of a study to measure the shape of the dose–effect curve, or to detect a threshold effect at the much lower dose levels which arise from natural environmental exposure. Lubin and Gail (1990) explored the requirements for a case–control study to discover whether the relationship between natural exposure to radon and an excess of lung cancer was linear or curved. They calculated that this would require 24 054 cases of lung cancer! (A cohort study, of course, would have been far more demanding.) Who could disagree with their conclusion that '... these calculations suggest that an epidemiologic study of this disease (phenomenon) is not feasible'? They continued, 'Enormous numbers of subjects are required, because of the small difference between the null and alternative hypotheses'. If this is the difficulty in merely distinguishing between a straight line and a curve, one must accept the total impossibility of plotting the actual values for a curve, or for identifying whether a step or threshold occurs at very low levels of exposure; yet this is precisely what we would need to know in order to have a firm scientific basis for public health policy on this major issue.

The conclusion is disheartening. Having argued that choice of the right control policy depends on knowing which of the situations in Fig. 3.1 really applies, it must now be admitted that this critical question is often unanswerable. When we announced our conclusions from the Atomic Energy Authority study at a press conference, the reporters at once asked, 'When are you going to get the real answer? What more research should be done?' Neither the media nor the public have grasped the fact that some critically important questions are unanswerable, either now or in the foreseeable future. We all need to learn how to live with uncertainty, including the scientific experts and the policy-makers. Unfortunately humankind cannot bear much uncertainty.

Needles in haystacks

Occupational exposure to vinyl chloride monomer causes haemangiosarcoma of the liver. This tumour is rare in the absence of that particular exposure, and this made it easy to detect the association. The situation would have been quite different if haemangiosarcoma had been a common tumour; the dangerous consequence of occupational exposure might have been just the same, but it would have been lost in the haystack of other cases.

Suppose that we take the background incidence of a disease to be unity (i.e. 1), but in people exposed to an uncommon but potent cause the incidence rises by 9, so that the new level is now 10. Thus the incidence of the disease has risen 10-fold and a case-control study should readily identify the problem. Suppose now that the background incidence were not 1 but 50; with just the same absolute excess (i.e. 9), due to our potent but uncommon cause, we should now have an incidence of 59, which implies a relative risk of less than 1.2. The public health problem is just the same as before but it has effectively become undetectable, for it is hard to think of any instance where a relative risk of less than about 1.5 has been identified as causal in the absence of other evidence. It is not just a problem of statistical power, which might be overcome in a larger study, but rather that of a true and important effect being lost to sight when it is surrounded by larger neighbours.

Suppose (and it is mere supposition) that the fluoridation of water supplies were to increase the incidence of gastric cancer by 1 per cent;

then this would imply about 100 attributable deaths in Britain each year. Such an increase would be undetectable. We are bad at identifying, and hence also bad at controlling, a hazard which modestly increases the frequency of an already common problem, in contrast with one which has a unique and therefore conspicuous result.

Illogically, this difference in detectability is matched by an opposite difference in its customary valuation. If a problem is common and has been around for a long time, then people come to accept it even if it is large; it is the exceptional or new which causes alarm. The toll of deaths from road traffic accidents vastly exceeds that from crashing aeroplanes, but only the latter lead to public inquiries. The seriousness of man-made sources of radiation as a cause of cancers is widely down-rated (especially by the radiation industry) because the total exposure from natural radiation is so much larger. This is illogical. If I break my leg, my problem is no less simply because a thousand others are similarly afflicted: the size of a problem is the size that it is, and each hazard needs to be considered in its own right.

Small but widespread risks: a public health disaster?

Having considered the situation of an uncommon exposure to a serious risk, we turn now to its opposite, namely the situation where many are exposed to an individually small risk.

People do not worry each time that they get into their motor cars, because the risk of an accident on that particular day is negligible. How low must a risk be before it can be regarded as negligible? Seemingly this is a matter more of perception than of statistics, for after passing a serious accident on a motorway most drivers slow down for a while, or a smoker may decide to give up because a close acquaintance has developed lung cancer. This suggests that, to be effective, health education may need to sharpen perception rather than simply convey information. It then soon runs into a limitation, for a risk which has not materialized within the individual's own experience is unlikely to be regarded seriously.

This pragmatic attitude protects us from perpetual anxiety and at the same time gives priority to experience over theory. Sensible though this attitude may be, it is extremely bad news for our hopes of improving public health. Because so many people drive their cars every day and nearly all return home safely, no one really expects to have an accident on any particular occasion. Therefore few feel any personal responsibility for the major problem of death and injury on the roads. The existence of the problem is recognized, but it is theoretical and remote rather than personal.

The usual response is to concentrate efforts on a high-risk subgroup where the risk is not negligible, such as drinking drivers (for road accidents), those with high blood cholesterol (for coronary heart disease), older mothers (for Down syndrome), workers and others exposed to excessive levels of radiation (for possible induction of cancers), and so on. This is a much more saleable message, because everyone can see that the risk is not so remote. This approach is not to be faulted for what it attempts but only for what it fails to confront, namely the public health problem arising from a small but widespread risk.

The cholesterol problem

Figure 3.2 has been assembled from data on the world's largest cohort study, which recorded mortality among the 361 662 men who were examined in order to determine their eligibility for the Multiple Risk Factor Intervention Trial (Martin *et al.* 1986). The figure shows three things. First, the bar diagram presents the distribution of serum cholesterol levels at the initial examination, the commonest values being around 5–5.5 mmol/l (194–213 mg/dl). Next, the broken curve shows how the incidence of fatal heart attacks rises steeply with increasing levels of cholesterol: at the highest level, about one man in 50 had died of a heart attack who would have been alive if he had had the risk of a low-cholesterol contemporary. This level of personal risk could not be considered negligible, but happily the prevalence of such an exposure is only 2 per cent.

This is the traditional or individual-centred approach to epidemiology, but we can also look at the problem for the population as a whole. The actual 6 year death rate from coronary heart disease was 7.3 per 1000. If, instead, all had experienced the much smaller rate of the low-cholesterol men (only a little over 3 per 1000), then coronary deaths would have been halved. This represents the total size of the

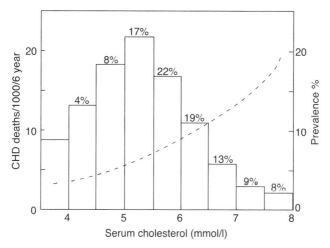

Fig. 3.2 Prevalence distribution (bars) of serum cholesterol concentration related to age-adjusted mortality from coronary heart disease (CHD) (broken curve) in men aged 40–59 years. The number above each bar is the percentage of the deaths 'attributable' to the cholesterol effect and arising at that level. (Data from Martin *et al.* 1986).

cholesterol-related problem for the whole population. We can now enquire how this total is distributed across the cholesterol range, and this is shown by the values at the heads of the bars in Fig. 3.2. A striking and highly important finding now emerges. The problem that was so worrying for the high-cholesterol individuals accounts for only 8 per cent of the total of fatal heart attacks that are statistically attributable to the cholesterol factor. The personal risk may be high, but fortunately this level of exposure involves relatively few people. By far the greater part of the problem arises from the zone that is around and a little above the centre of the distribution. The personal excess risk here is small, and to the individual it might even be seen as negligible (only about one fatal chance in 300), but so many people are exposed to it that collectively the effect is large.

This illustrates one of the most fundamental axioms in preventive medicine: *a large number of people exposed to a small risk may generate many more cases than a small number exposed to a high risk.* Wherever this axiom applies, it means that a high-risk preventive strategy is dealing only with the margin of the problem, and it can improve its achievement only by extending its coverage; in the cholesterol example, even an extension to half the population would still fail to touch a substantial portion of the attributable cases. Where there is mass exposure to risk (even to low level risk), there is a need for mass measures of control. And that means that some way must be found to reduce the risk of large numbers of people who, more often than not, will not benefit from the change (the 'prevention paradox' (see p. 47)).

There can be a conflict here between the collective interest, which requires community-wide change, and that of many of the individuals concerned, who could well consider that their prospect of benefit was negligible. (The concept of 'negligible benefit' is the counterpart of 'negligible risk', and it raises the same issues (see p. 57)). It is like a lottery in which the prize may be glitteringly large, but if the chance of winning it is too remote then people may not be bothered to enter. The health prize may be the difference between life and death, but if the statistical chance that it will affect any particular individual is too small and remote, then people may not want to bother. However, only if they choose to bother can prevention be effective.

'A touch of depression'

To a doctor, depression means a diagnosis, and a diagnosis splits off a distinct group of deviants needing treatment from the 'normal' population, who ought not to be treated. In common speech and experience the meaning is much wider, for at some time or another nearly everyone feels a bit depressed, but medical and lay people alike would agree with the physician in *Macbeth* (Act 5, Scene 3) that 'in such matters the patient must minister to himself'.

Epidemiological research into depression employs standardized inventories of symptoms whose results are then combined to yield a score. It might be thought natural to use this score in order to characterize each individual's position on the continuum from 'not at all depressed' to 'suicidal', much as intelligence tests are used to give each person an IQ score, but this is not what psychiatric researchers do. Instead, they prefer to define an arbitrary score, corresponding to the level above which they are likely to recognize the individual as 'a case for treatment'; they then report the prevalence of such cases, rarely displaying any interest in the wide spread of scores below this arbitrary level. This has restricted our knowledge of the mental health of populations (Rose 1989).

There have been a few notable exceptions. Figure 3.3 sets out (in the same format as Fig. 3.2) the findings of an American researcher (Brenner 1985). The depression inventory used in this survey recorded the presence of each of the relevant items (early morning waking, diurnal mood variation, etc.). The bars in the figure identify the proportion of people reporting various numbers of positive items. Conventionally, the presence of six or more of these items is considered to identify individuals whom a psychiatrist is likely to call 'cases of depression'; however, as with blood pressure (Fig. 2.1) and serum cholesterol (Fig. 3.2), it seems that nature does not recognize any sharp split between 'well' and 'sick' (the peak for the group with six or more items is due simply to aggregation of all the higher classes).

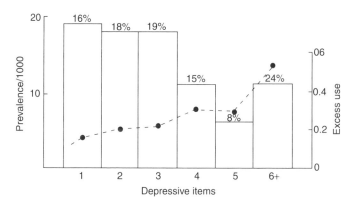

Fig. 3.3 Findings in a population survey of depression showing (1) the prevalence of reporting of various numbers of depressive features (bars), related to (2) the excess use of social supports above the rate for 'no depressive features' (broken line) and to (3) the proportions of this total excess attributable to different levels of depression (numbers above bars).

Does 'a touch of depression' matter? Brenner tried to answer this question by relating the depression score to the probability of using social supports (shown by the broken line in the figure). Clearly the answer is 'yes', for the use of supports increases with every step up the depression scale. Using this measure it appears that those with just two positive items are functionally worse off than those with a single positive item, even though both are far removed from anything that would be called 'a case of depression'. What Fig. 3.2 showed for the spectrum of a risk factor (cholesterol) is now seen also to apply to the spectrum of a measure of health outcome: it is better to be very healthy than averagely healthy.

This expresses the findings from Brenner's study as they apply to individuals. What do they imply for the burden on the community? This is indicated by the numbers at the top of the bars in Fig. 3.3, which show the proportion of the total of depression-related disability which arose at each level of depression score. The conspicuously disabled high scorers (the 'cases') accounted for only a quarter of the excess community burden, whereas most of the disability came from the large number of people around the middle of the distribution, and one-third arose among those who reported only one or two positive items. 'A touch of depression' is mildly disappointing news for the affected individuals but it is bad news for the community. Prevention, to be effective, must address the whole range of the problem.

Conclusions

Two issues concerning the shape of the dose–effect relationship are critical for preventive policy. How much of the burden of ill health is compressed within an identifiable group where high exposure carries a high personal risk? Is there an exposure threshold below which risk is negligible and can be ignored?

Both these questions require us to look at the whole ranges of both exposure to causes and health outcomes. Where research has proceeded in this way, it has often appeared that there is a graded threshold-free relation between cause and effect, and where this applies, it is common to find that the burden of ill health comes more from the many who are exposed to a low inconspicuous risk than from the few who face an obvious problem. This sets a limit to the effectiveness of an individual (high-risk) approach to prevention.

In practice, research studies may lack the size and power to be able to tell whether or not a threshold effect exists, or to indicate how much benefit can be expected from reducing the exposure to a widespread low-level risk. Preventive medicine, like the rest of medicine, should be as scientific as possible, but we should not expect to find more than a few islands of firm ground, and for the rest we must learn to live with uncertainty and to be satisfied with best judgements. Most decisions on health policy are provisional, and they are subject to review in the light of experience and new ideas.

Chapter 4

Prevention for individuals and the 'high-risk' strategy

Illness is a personal and not a collective event: it happens to individuals, and statistics mislead by presenting only the totals. According to recent World Health Organization reports, covering 56 of the world's populations, annual deaths from lung cancer numbered 471 434 (nearly all preventable). What this really means is that there were $1 + 1 + 1 + 1 \ldots$ etc. individuals, each of whom suffered severe personal distress. The objective of preventive medicine is the avoidance of a series of individual misfortunes, and so it is natural to believe that preventive action should be targeted on the individuals at risk.

In all societies the doctor's primary role is seen as the care of sick individuals, and young people who choose to enter medicine do so with this picture in their minds. For most, their subsequent professional ethos will be founded on accepting responsibility for patients. Indeed, in some specialities this individual-centred approach is so dominant as to exclude almost completely any other view of health problems, for example in surgery and psychiatry.

This priority of concern for action at the level of needy individuals also receives wide support from outside medicine. Charitable organizations for the relief of famine and other kinds of distress know that fund-raising appeals are best accompanied by a picture, preferably named, of a person in need, preferably a child. It is much harder to raise support for collective action against the underlying causes of a problem, because the public's perception of need is in personal terms. Similarly, politicians and governments favour action confined to a needy minority rather than any recognition that health could reflect national or social policies. They argue that individuals, with support from their doctors, should be held responsible for their own health.

Thus among doctors, public, and governments alike the natural focus for preventive medicine is action for individuals.

Prevention and clinical care

Just as in an enlightened penal system the treatment of offenders is seen as an opportunity to make future offences less likely, so also in medicine the clinician who treats a sick person has an opportunity to use the occasion for prevention as well as cure. Every doctor who sees a patient should be asking, 'Why did this illness occur? What can be done to reduce the risk of recurrence?'

An American survey to discover why people stop smoking found that the commonest reply was 'Because my physician advised it'. The medical consultation can provide an effective opening for prevention. The timing is right, since patient and doctor alike recognize that there is a problem whose recurrence they wish to avoid. The consultation also provides a natural opportunity to initiate preventive action, needing no extra organization or staff. It is unfortunate that many consultations are still dominated by short-term thoughts of treatment, to the exclusion of a concern for future health. Lack of time is a serious problem, but the underlying implication is that a diversion of time from treatment to prevention would not be worthwhile. Tudor Hart has written

Prevention is still seen as an essentially administrative task … requiring few clinical skills, performed at the expense of demand-led response to symptomatic disease. (Hart 1990)

The situation is changing rapidly, notably in general practice. Indeed, there is some danger of prevention being oversold. Preventive measures which could bring real health benefits are available to general practitioners, but the list is at present a short one and the evidence for enlarging it should be no less clear than that required before we accept a new therapy into routine practice.

Some of the preventive options available to doctors are a natural extension of their familiar clinical skills (for example, screening and immunization), but many involve counselling (for example, management of problems relating to alcohol, diet, or stress) and here the requisite skills lie outside the regular medical range. It remains to be discovered how many doctors would acquire such skills and enjoy using them, if they had appropriate training. For those who are oriented by temperament towards the more authoritarian approach of acute medical care, the task will need to be deputed to a trained nurse or other health counsellor.

The high-risk strategy

Action for individuals commonly implies first some means of identifying those in special need, i.e. those who are at special risk, and in clinical practice this commonly means some form of screening assessment. Preventive action may then take one of two forms, either controlling the level of exposure to a cause (for example, reducing house dust and house dust mites in homes with an asthmatic child) or providing protection against the effects of exposure in order to forestall complications (for example, hepatitis vaccine for those with an occupational risk).

Some illustrations of the widespread interest in this strategy, embracing most specialities, are given in Table 4.1. In these examples, each of the risk factors is measured as a continuous score. The distribution is then dichotomized in order to identify a 'high-risk' group comprising those individuals who qualify for special attention; the remainder are classed as 'normal' and can be left in peace (see p. 43). As with clinical diagnosis, this arbitrary dichotomy is an operational necessity. Whether the aim is to reduce the level of exposure to a cause or to control some intermediate variable, like blood pressure, the theoretical hope is a truncation of the risk factor distribution (Fig. 4.1) in order to relieve the high-risk status of the deviant minority without interfering with the rest of the population.

Motivation

The strong attraction of the high-risk preventive strategy is that intervention is matched to the needs of the individual. This makes sense to patient and adviser alike. In our controlled trial of anti-smoking advice (Rose *et al.* 1982) we first undertook medical examinations of nearly 20 000 middle-aged male civil servants (the Whitehall Study). Smoking is of course a health risk to everyone, but we recalled only those smokers whose examination had given evidence of exceptional

Table 4.1 Examples of continuous risk factors and related health outcomes

Speciality	Risk factor	Outcome to be prevented
General medicine	Blood pressure	Stroke
	Body weight	Diabetes
Infectious diseases	Occupational exposure to blood	Hepatitis
Paediatrics	'APGAR' score	Neonatal death
	Risk score	'Sudden infant death'
Cardiology	Blood cholesterol	Coronary heart attack
Obstetrics	Maternal age etc.	Down syndrome*
	Blood pressure	Toxaemia
Surgery	Oestrogen receptor status	Breast cancer
Orthopaedics	Osteoporosis	Fracture
Ophthalmology	Intraocular pressure	Glaucoma
Occupational medicine	Blood lead	Lead poisoning
Environmental medicine	Exposure to lead	Intellectual defect
Social services	Risk score	Child abuse

* For the community this may indeed prevent the appearance of cases, but for the fetus involved it is suppressive rather than preventive medicine!

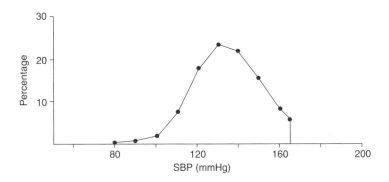

Fig. 4.1 The ideal outcome of a high-risk preventive strategy: truncation of the distribution. (Data for systolic blood pressure (SBP) in middle-aged men).

risk and we explained to them individually why they in particular would benefit from stopping smoking. The result was that more than half gave up cigarettes, usually immediately. This compares with success rates of around 10 per cent from routinely given antismoking advice, and it shows that matching the advice to the individual can induce powerful motivation.

Health professionals much prefer to confine their efforts to people who clearly need them. 'Why me?' and 'Why now?' are the natural responses of those who are told that a lifetime habit should be changed, especially if they feel perfectly well at the time. In the high-risk approach, no advice is given except where there is a ready answer to these questions.

Identifying risk: screening

Screening was developed as a means of identifying early disease, such as mass radiography to detect tuberculosis, with the objective of earlier and perhaps more effective treatment. This amounts to an extension of the range of therapeutics, but here we are concerned only with preventive medicine, aimed at forestalling the first onset of disease by detecting risk factors such as those listed in Table 4.1. These represent the harbingers of future trouble rather than actual disease.

The information required for risk assessment may sometimes require no special search, as when it is based on maternal age or occupational exposure, because these can be identified from routine records. In contrast, multiple problems of ethics, organization, and expense arise when healthy people are summoned to a medical examination.

Screening examinations can be popular, particularly if they include an X-ray or some other impressive piece of high-technology apparatus handled by a specialist team. This popularity indicates a widespread lack of confidence in personal health and a fear of the future. Our own studies gave a strong impression that most of those who attend are seeking, not the discovery of hidden troubles, but rather a reassurance that they have no unusual problems. Such reassurance is regarded as a guarantee of good health, at least for a year or so, and it restores some confidence in the future. To the public this represents an important benefit.

The classic paper by Wilson and Jungner (1968) set out the policy guidelines for screening to detect early disease. Some additional principles and caveats relating to examinations aimed at risk assessment are given below.

Policy guidelines for screening to assess risk

1 *There should be no screening without adequate resources for advice and long-term care* Unlike the examination of a sick patient, a screening examination is usually a medical initiative to which the subjects are urged to respond. If the findings are negative then no ethical difficulty is raised; however, someone who is told of a health problem, previously unsuspected, suffers distress which may persist.

The possibility that continued support may relieve this distress was demonstrated in the Medical Research Council trial of hypertension screening and treatment for hypertension. Anthony Mann, an epidemiological psychiatrist, assessed the mental health of participants when they attended for screening examinations and then again at intervals over the next year (Mann 1977). He found a significant improvement in psychiatric morbidity during this period among those who entered the trial and received continuing care, but this was not seen among those whose screening results did not qualify them for trial entry.

This provides the first reason why screening ought not to be introduced unless those found to have a problem can receive personal and expert interpretation and advice. Fear has been aroused, often inappropriately, and an escape route must if possible be indicated. 'Supermarket' or 'pharmacy shop' screening is to be deprecated.

A further reason to link screening with professional care is that in the absence of such care it is likely to be ineffective. Health education research suggests that information by itself may have little influence on behaviour; it needs to be accompanied by some personal challenge, guidance, and continuing support and interest. Indeed, the success of the whole effort may be proportional to the staff time that can be made available, and to the training and skill of the health advisers.

The appropriate duration of support depends on the circumstances, and in particular on whether the advice or treatment requires some continuing effort by the subjects. In the World Health

Organization European collaborative trial of heart disease prevention (World Health Organization European Collaborative Group 1986) we had to withdraw our personal contacts with participants after 4 years because of exhaustion of our funds. The men had been encouraged to change their life-style, which meant being different from their friends and workmates in their habits of eating, smoking, and exercise. When support from the trial staff ceased they were drawn back into the 'normal' behaviour of their society; their earlier improvement in risk factors was quickly lost, and with it they soon also lost all the reduced incidence of heart disease which had previously been achieved.

This illustrates how a preventive policy which requires sustained and effortful personal changes, whether in life-style or by taking medication, is at a great disadvantage in comparison with the 'one-off' effort of immunization or the benefits derived passively from environmental changes. Unfortunately, the requirement that a minority must act differently from the majority tends to be inherent in the high-risk preventive strategy, and this limits its effectiveness.

Since the success of screening depends on after-care, and since this may need to be maintained for years, it follows that a policy of mass screening for risk identification presupposes a medical care system which is able to provide continuity of long-term personal care for everyone. This is a major obstacle to effective preventive care in countries, such as the USA, which lack a general practitioner system covering the whole population. In Britain, and in other countries fortunate enough to possess such a system, at least the potential is there for long-term personal preventive care, but its realization requires a substantial additional investment in staff, training, and organization. Most countries are still seeking for the right way to reward the medical team for providing preventive services.

2 *Selective screening and care are more cost effective than mass screening* Simple and readily available information may often indicate that risk is more likely to be found in one group than another. This can make it profitable to plan a two-stage process in which one looks for high-risk individuals only within a high-risk sector of the population.

Table 4.2 gives an example of some estimates we made of the potential benefits of screening for blood (serum) cholesterol and of the

Table 4.2 Estimates of potential reduction in coronary heart disease deaths from screening for raised serum cholesterol (>6.5 mmol/l) in different age and sex groups

	Age (years)			
	25–34	**35–44**	**45–54**	**55–64**
Percentage with raised level				
Men	20	35	40	45
Women	15	20	50	70
5 year deaths per 1000 in this group				
Men	1.2	5.8	21.3	48.1
Women	0.2	1.1	4.5	15.9
No. screened to prevent 1 death in 5 years*				
Men	21 100	2500	600	230
Women	137 300	23 200	2200	450
No. treated for 5 years to prevent 1 death*				
Men	4200	860	230	100
Women	20 600	4650	1100	320

* Assuming 20% reduction in deaths among all eligibles.

efforts that would be required to achieve them (Khaw and Rose 1989). The absolute size of benefits depends on the particular assumptions in the model, but this would not affect the main conclusions.

The table shows that the death rate associated with raised cholesterol—and with it, the potential for preventive benefit—increases steeply with age, and at each age it is higher in men than in women. This produces some startling differences in the effort and costs involved in preventing one fatal heart attack through a 5 year programme. For men aged 55–64 this involves screening about 230 people, followed by 100 'treatment-years' of advice. Relative to other preventive or therapeutic measures this would be reckoned as good value. In complete contrast, the prevention of one death over a 5 year period in women aged 25–34 would involve screening more than 130 000, followed by more than 20 000 person-years of treatment—worse by a factor in excess of 200. Unless one takes the extreme and wholly unrealistic view that the saving of a life is worth any price at all, then it is hard to justify asking young women to come for a cholesterol measurement, and, since we lack the resources for giving personal and long-term support to everyone, it is surely better to concentrate it on those who are mostly likely to benefit.

Costs and efficiency are not, of course, the sole guide to policy. General practitioners who allowed only men to have access to a popular service might find themselves in trouble! They would also be missing one of the indirect benefits of the high-risk policy, namely a spill-over of interest and information to family and friends.

The findings in Table 4.2 have to be seen against a background of growing pressures to measure everyone's blood cholesterol. Indeed, the American policy is that we should all 'know our cholesterol number', and, quite arbitrarily, a figure of 6.5 mmol/l has been defined by expert bodies as the limit beyond which individual advice is called for. The implications of this recommendation have not been thought through, since this definition of the high-risk group might currently include up to 70 per cent of women past the age of 55 years. Of course, the higher the prevalence of 'high-risk' status, the greater the potential benefits to the community from treating all those at high risk, but total costs rise disproportionately and the policy starts to lose all meaning if it has to embrace a large part of the population.

3 *The purpose is to assess reversible risk—not risk factors* Health service managers and policy-makers are often, quite rightly, castigated for being preoccupied with process and ignoring the health outcomes of the service. They see a 'good' health service as one that supports many activities, such as surgical operations and other treatments, at minimum costs. 'This has been a good year for the National Health Service', the minister wrote in his annual report, 'we have treated more patients than ever before'. Those who manage health services according to the principles of the market are particularly prone to such folly.

Clinicians are not exempt from this blinkered attitude, for they often judge the success of a treatment by its effects on the investigations.

'The treatment was successful and the patient's test results returned to normal. (Unfortunately, he died)'.

The analogous error arises in a common but mistaken view of the purpose of risk assessment by screening. The real purpose should be to identify those people in whom intervention offers the most benefit. Thus the measurement of a particular risk factor is but one step on the road to assessing overall risk, and that is only an intermediary to the possibility of risk reduction. Health services and all their activities are concerned with one thing only, and that is health. Everything else must be judged by its contribution to that goal (Cochrane 1972).

This perspective has several implications. First, the excess risk associated with a particular factor may depend on its context, and hence it can only be judged in relation to other relevant characteristics of the individual. The risk associated with household radon depends heavily on the smoking habits of the residents. Non-smokers have little to fear from radon in their houses.

A similar multiplicative interaction is seen between smoking and the hazards of asbestos exposure (Table 4.3). The relative risk of lung cancer associated with exposure is similar in smokers and non-smokers (about fivefold in each instance). Relative risk measures causal force, and often (as here) is generalizable across different groups or populations. This makes it the researcher's preferred measure of risk, but it is a highly misleading guide to policy, quite failing here to identify the smoker's far higher absolute increment of risk when he is also exposed to asbestos. Policy decisions must therefore be founded on absolute, not relative, risk estimates, and they should take account of those other factors which modify the risk of a particular exposure.

Table 4.3 The relative risks of death from lung cancer according to exposure to asbestos and cigarette smoking

| | | Cigarettes | |
		No	Yes
Asbestos	No	1.0	10.9
	Yes	5.2	53.2

Nowhere is this concept more important than in cardiovascular risk screening. The usual guidelines for action often consider risk factors one at a time, each in isolation from the others, and they then lay down a particular value above which an intervention is prescribed. For example, in the case of cholesterol, this may be 'more than 6.5 mmol/l' or for diastolic pressure, 'more than 100 mmHg'. This provides a poor guide to the individual's risk of suffering a heart attack, as can be seen from Fig. 4.2.

The results in this figure are taken from a mammoth-sized American study in which 361 662 men were screened in order to determine their eligibility for the Multiple Risk Factor Intervention Trial. Their risk factor levels were then related to mortality in the ensuing 6 years (Martin *et al.* 1986). The risk of death from coronary heart disease, indicated by the height of each column, is presented in relation to various combinations of three risk factors: smoking, blood pressure, and blood cholesterol, with the last two having been classified into thirds of their distributions. Following conventional screening practice, everyone with a cholesterol value in the upper third would be classified in a similar 'high-risk' category. This simplistic approach conceals gross inequalities of excess risk. For example, the excess (expressed in relation to the minimum risk group—the non-smokers with low blood pressure and low cholesterol) ranges from 5.6 (7.2–1.6) in non-smokers with low blood pressure up to 13.0 (14.6–1.6) in smokers with raised pressure. Thus the significance of one and the same cholesterol result may be more than doubled according to the context in which it finds itself. (The range would be greater still if one also took account of age and sex.)

These examples tell us that risk assessment must consider all relevant factors together rather than confine attention to a single test, for nearly all diseases are multifactorial.

Earlier in this chapter (p. 72) an attempt was made to compare the potential benefits of cholesterol screening and intervention in different groups, in particular younger women and older men. The risks in the absence of any intervention have been reasonably well established, but in order to estimate the benefits of action it was necessary to make an assumption about the effectiveness of treatment, and this assumption rested on guesswork, not evidence. This is a common problem. Risk may be readily identifiable, but our ability to reduce

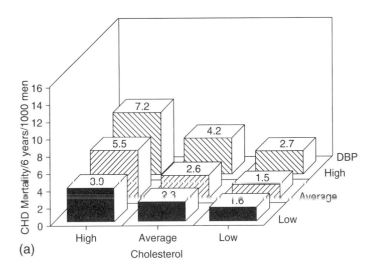

(a)

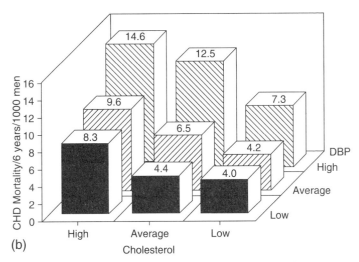

(b)

Fig. 4.2 Coronary heart disease (CHD) mortality in middle-aged American men according to their levels of blood cholesterol and diastolic blood pressure (DBP) in (a) non-smokers and (b) smokers.

the risk by consequent action (which is what really needs to be known) depends on three factors:

- effective advice or treatment;
- resources to offer it to those who need advice or treatment;
- acceptance of advice or treatment and (generally) long-term implementation.

The first of these calls for controlled trials whose outcome measure is disease. The second requires that the skills and resources which were available in the trials, usually in 'centres of excellence', should also be available generally and under ordinary service conditions. The third depends on the response of the people concerned and on their opportunities to act on the advice offered; for life-style changes, this acceptance of change needs to be assessed over many years. Such information may only become available long after the decision to adopt the policy.

Clearly, the estimates of benefit, crucial though they are, may suffer from wide limits of uncertainty, and more research may be called for in relation to each of these three key factors. Action and continuing research can legitimately go ahead side by side, even though the research may finally show that the action was mistaken. It is unrealistic to demand proof or certainty before action, and a demand for more research can be just an excuse for avoiding difficult decisions.

In summary, the purpose of risk assessment is not to categorize individuals according to a test result nor even as to their overall risk, but rather to identify those who can be helped, or helped most, by preventive action. A wrong approach may select the wrong people.

Strengths of the high-risk preventive strategy

An approach to preventive medicine which focuses its efforts on needy individuals, and which utilizes the established framework of the medical services, clearly has attractions (US Preventive Services Task Force 1989; Rose 1990*a*). Some of the principal merits of a high-risk strategy are discussed below.

1 *Intervention is appropriate to the individual* The high-risk preventive strategy is the natural outcome of that branch of aetiological research which deals with the causes of disease in individuals

(Rose 1985). Nowadays the commonest type of epidemiological enquiry is the case–control study, whose purpose is to discover how sick and healthy individuals differ. Most cohort studies are concerned to identify risk factors, again in order to answer that fundamental question: 'Why did *this* person become sick, whilst others remain well?'

Establishing the risk factors and causes of disease in individuals may permit the action to be matched to the individual's special need or problem. Thus the diabetic mother in particular is urged to control her obesity during pregnancy, salt restriction is recommended for the man with hypertension, and the smoker with impaired ventilatory function is urged to give up cigarettes. It makes sense that advice should in this way be appropriate to the individual; this appeals both to the individual and the doctor, and their motivation is enhanced.

2 *It avoids interference with those who are not at special risk* Since most diseases involve only a minority, it follows that in theory most people need not be troubled with preventive measures–if only we knew who were heading for disease! In practice, of course, the majority can be given only a qualified reassurance, but still, the cautious teetotal driver of a Volvo car is at relatively small risk of a fatal accident, just as a non-smoker blessed with a serum cholesterol of only 4 mmol/l is at relatively low risk of a heart attack. To urge preventive action on those who have small prospect of benefit does not make much sense, and if its implementation involves disturbance, cost, or (especially) risk, then it may be bad advice. The high-risk preventive strategy avoids getting into such a situation (although it should be realized that differences in need are commonly a matter of degree— there is no absolute distinction between the high-risk and population strategies).

3 *It is readily accommodated within the ethos and organization of medical care* A man goes to see his doctor complaining, say, of a pain in his neck. The doctor takes the opportunity to check his blood pressure, which is found to be raised. It remains raised at two further visits, and the doctor then tells him that he is 'suffering from hypertension'. Next there follow the giving and receiving of a prescription, which witnesses to a new contract

between them: henceforward the man is regarded for the rest of his life as 'a patient', accommodated within the familiar medical care organization. In fact he is not a patient at all, as his hypertensive care is a matter of prevention and not therapeutics, but the doctor has little difficulty in blurring the distinction between 'patients' and 'almost-patients'. The man himself will probably accept this, at least in Western cultures. In contrast, in African and Asian cultures it is common to regard treatment as being needed only for those who feel ill.

The acceptance of a preventive responsibility by clinicians brings great advantages. It helps to bridge the separation of clinical services and public health, and from a simple extension of normal clinical care there may grow a broader interest in preventive activities. It is surely better to keep prevention within the mainstream of medicine than to encourage a new speciality of 'preventive medicine'.

4 *It offers a cost-effective use of resources* Medical resources cannot stretch to providing personal preventive care and long-term support to everyone, even if that were desirable. This necessarily implies a system of rationing, which should give priority to those who are either most likely to benefit or likely to benefit most.

One of the painful lessons from health education has been that once-only advice can be a waste of time. Many doctors are disillusioned by their efforts to get fat patients to lose weight, a disappointment commonly shared by their patients. Often there has been little more than a firm admonition to lose weight, perhaps accompanied by a diet sheet, and the course of events was not thereby changed. A few, but only a few, have reported a better outcome. Sustained success in this difficult area seems to require considerable effort on both sides, including a proper assessment of current eating habits, a mutually agreed plan or 'contract', and continuing support. Given this investment, worthwhile progress may be possible (e.g. Stamler *et al.* 1984). Clearly such help cannot be offered to everyone who is overweight: to be cost-effective, it must be focused on those to whom it is most important (such as those with hypertension or diabetes).

5 *Selectivity improves the benefit-to-risk ratio* Every intervention must carry some costs and a possibility of adverse effects. If the costs

and risks are much the same for everybody, then the ratio of benefits to costs will be more favourable where the benefits are larger.

Amniocentesis is necessary in order to make a diagnosis of Down syndrome. Unfortunately, it occasionally provokes abortion of a normal fetus, and this must be balanced against the benefit of obtaining a correct diagnosis. It is widely concluded that the risk is only justifiable in a high-risk pregnancy (i.e. in an older mother, and after non-invasive biochemical tests of alpha-fetoprotein, unconjugated oestriol, and human gonadotrophins have proved positive (Wald *et al.* 1988)).

The use of medications may offer an attractive short cut to prevention. Although rejected by many as 'unnatural', to others they represent a more impressive—and perhaps also less painful—weapon than simple changes in life-style. Sometimes there may be no adequate substitute, as when aspirin and beta-blockers are given in order to ward off a recurrence of myocardial infarction, but there are powerful pressures towards overuse. Doctors may find it easier to write a prescription than to counsel, their patients may be more satisfied, and the highly influential pharmaceutical companies are delighted.

The necessity for selectivity in the long-term use of drugs for preventive purposes was first demonstrated by the World Health Organization's trial of the drug clofibrate, used at that time for reducing the blood cholesterol level (Committee of Principal Investigators 1980). Until that trial it was widely agreed that at least this drug was safe. The trial showed that it does indeed prevent heart attacks, but unfortunately there were about one-third more deaths among those receiving clofibrate than among the placebo-treated control patients. The excess deaths were not due to any conspicuous cause, and the effect could never have been detected other than by a very large controlled trial (actually 208 000 man-years). The risk was estimated at only one excess death per 1000 treatment-years.

The lesson from this trial is important: *the long-term use of drugs in prevention is justified only within a high-risk group.* We have no means of excluding a level of risk which, however small for the individual, might exceed overall the hoped for benefit—except where that benefit is known to be substantial. This effectively rules out any mass use of long-term drugs, especially since trials rarely continue for longer than about 5 years, leaving us quite in the dark concerning lifetime effects. It is only in individuals known to be at exceptional risk that such uncertainty may be acceptable.

Weaknesses of the high-risk preventive strategy

1 *Prevention becomes medicalized* To be preoccupied with health is unhealthy. The man who went to see his doctor because he had a pain in his neck walked away from that encounter bearing a label 'hypertensive patient', which he must now wear for the rest of his life. Having hitherto perceived himself as healthy, he now has to see himself as someone needing to take pills and to see the doctor regularly. He was, he thought, normal; now he is a patient. This may be unavoidable and justified by the benefits, but it is a major cost.

The effects of 'labelling' should constitute a prominent item in the balance-sheet by which a screening policy is assessed, but they have received all too little attention. Many authoritative policy reviews show no awareness that the problem even exists (for example, an official British statement on blood cholesterol testing by the Standing Medical Advisory Committee (1990), policy statements on screening for cervical cancer, etc.).

It is difficult to quantify the mental trauma resulting from 'labelling', and attempts to do so have been few. However, one such attempt was made in the Medical Research Council hypertension trial (Mann 1977) (see p. 70): participants answered the General Health Questionnaire, followed by a standard psychiatric interview. Although the results were broadly reassuring, a serious doubt must remain as to whether these methods, which were developed as a means of detecting mental illness, are appropriate for measuring mental trauma to normal people.

The danger of making this sort of assumption was demonstrated rather dramatically by Rosenhan's famous study 'On being sane in insane places' (Rosenhan 1973). In his experiment eight sane people feigned a single hallucinatory experience. They were duly seen by psychiatrists and all were admitted to mental hospitals, where they remained for periods ranging from 7 to 52 days. Whilst in hospital they behaved in a normal manner and were fully co-operative, but not a single psychiatrist recognized any of the subjects as sane! Thus standard techniques for identifying mental illness may be poor measures of 'labelling'-induced anxiety, impaired confidence, or altered self-image in normal people.

2 *Success is only palliative and temporary* Disease results when susceptible individuals are exposed to external causes. The high-risk preventive strategy seeks to help those individuals who are either unduly susceptible or unusually exposed, this help being directed either to protection against the effects of exposure (as by immunization or cholesterol-lowering drugs) or to reducing the individual's level of exposure (as by advice to drink less alcohol or a change in occupational exposure).

This approach to prevention does not seek to alter the situations which determine exposure, nor to attack the underlying reasons why the particular health problem exists: it simply offers protection to the most vulnerable individuals from the effects of a hazardous situation, which continues. This is analogous to famine relief, which feeds the hungry but does not tackle the causes of famine, or vaccinating a population against cholera rather than improving their water supply. The strategy may be lifesaving for the people concerned, but there will always be such vulnerable individuals and as long as the roots of the problem remain they will still need to be rescued. The achievements of the high-risk strategy, as of any individual-based approach, are limited to the individuals concerned: they are palliative, local, and temporary.

3 *The strategy is behaviourally inadequate* Eating, smoking, exercise, sexual practices, and other life-style characteristics are all substantially shaped and constrained by the norms of our particular society and by the behaviour of our peers. If we try to eat differently from our friends it will not only be inconvenient, but we risk being regarded as cranks or hypochondriacs, and anyway success will depend on the right foods being available, labelled where necessary with their nutrient content. If a man's work environment encourages heavy drinking (such as employment in the armed services), then to be told that this may damage his liver will probably have little effect. Advice which aims to reduce

HIV infection or cervical cancer by reducing the number of sexual contacts is unlikely to succeed as long as promiscuity is socially approved. Encouragement of leisure-time exercise will get little response as long as watching the television is regarded as the normal way to spend an evening, or if exercise facilities are not accessible, affordable, and attractive.

It is difficult for people to step out of line with their peers and workmates, yet that is what an individual or high-risk approach to prevention requires.

4 *It is limited by a poor ability to predict the future of individuals* It sounds impressive to say that a man with a high coronary risk score may be 20 or even 30 times as likely to suffer a heart attack as a man with a very low score, but if this man is considering the need to make radical changes in his life-style, then what he needs to know is some absolute measure of his chances, and by how much he could hope to improve them in the foreseeable future. Unfortunately the ability to estimate the average risk for a group, which may be good, is not matched by any corresponding ability to predict which individuals are going to fall ill soon.

This point emerged forcibly in the Medical Research Council trial of treatment for mild hypertension. The relative risk of a stroke increased steeply with rising blood pressure, and treatment effectively reduced it, but for any one individual the absolute risk was low, and overall it needed 850 person-years of treatment in order to prevent one stroke. Indeed, after 5 or 6 years in the trial, 95 per cent of those receiving only placebo tablets remained alive and well.

Figure 4.3 comes from our Whitehall Study of cardiovascular risk factors in London civil servants. It shows the distribution of blood pressures recorded at the initial screening examination, in men who survived during the following 18 years, comparing it with the distribution in those who died during this period from a heart attack or stroke. The contrast is distinctly unimpressive. There is a significant upward shift among those who were destined for trouble, but it is small (averaging less than 10 mmHg). It is on such differences that our recognition of important risk factors is based, but when the extent of overlap is considered, it is not surprising that an individual's

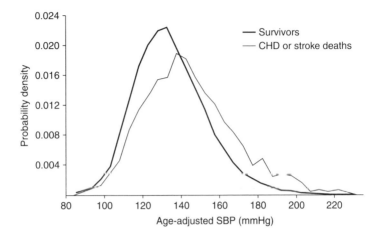

Fig. 4.3 The distribution of systolic blood pressure (SBP) in middle-aged men who died during the following 18 years from heart attack or stroke, compared with the distribution in survivors.

future is so often misassessed. 'Low-risk' individuals may fall sick, and most 'high-risk' individuals will stay well.

Table 4.4 illustrates the problem this raises for a preventive policy which is limited to those at high risk. It comes from the UK section of our heart disease prevention trial (World Health Organization

Table 4.4 Prediction of the risk of myocardial infarction in the next 5 years, based on the presence or absence of risk factors, with or without additional evidence of early heart disease (men aged 40–59 years).

Screening result	Percentage of men	Percentage later suffering an attack	Percentage of all attacks occurring in this group
All men	100	4	100
Elevated risk factors	15	7	32
Elevated risk factors + early disease	2	22	12

Source: Heller *et al*. 1984

European Collaborative Group 1986; Heller *et al.* 1984), and it examines the predictive ability of different definitions of 'high risk', as assessed by a simple examination which included the main coronary risk factors together with some measures of early heart disease (symptoms and electrocardiography). If 'high risk' were defined by elevated risk factors alone, then 15 per cent of men would have qualified for preventive help, but follow-up showed that only 7 per cent of these men actually developed serious trouble in the next 5 years, the other 93 per cent remaining well. Also, a preventive strategy confined to this group could only hope to influence one-third of future cases.

If a stricter criterion of high risk were to be adopted, requiring evidence of early disease as well as risk factors, then the size of the group to be advised falls drastically (down to 2 per cent of the study population). The risk to the men concerned is now much higher (22 per cent), but still nearly 80 per cent remained well, and from the community's point of view we are now considering a policy which has no chance at all of preventing 88 per cent of all heart attacks.

We are left with this impasse, reflecting the weakness of predictions when applied to individuals: if a high-risk group is defined broadly, then most of those included will not actually prove to have a problem, but if it is defined narrowly, it can contribute little towards reducing the total burden of disease. What is best for the selected individuals is worst for the community.

5 *Problems of feasibility and costs* At one extreme, these problems may be quite small. APGAR scores on new-born babes offer a quick and simple way to identify which ones need special care, for only one assessment is needed and the necessary care is completed relatively soon. At the other extreme the difficulties and costs may be formidable. Routine tonometry to detect raised intraocular pressure and risk of glaucoma has foundered as a policy because the test requires specialist skills, it is not popular with the participants, its predictive power is low, the treatment is incompletely effective, and long-term compliance is poor.

Many other policies would fall intermediately on a scale of difficulty and expense. Adequate evaluation of preventive policies has been exceptional, expressed in terms of the total costs (to service providers and participants) of preventing one 'critical event'. The best examples have been set for those measures which require only a single or other brief intervention, such as vaccines or vitamin K prophylaxis of haemorrhagic disease of the newborn.

One of the worst-evaluated policies (but one of the most popular) is blood cholesterol screening. There has been no adequate costing, nor can there be at present since we do not yet know the extent of compliance with dietary advice, either under average service conditions (which are quite different from those in special clinics) or over a period of many years. The promotion of screening has become badly out of step with the provision of trained staff to provide long-term support. There is commonly no clear policy on selectivity and priorities, whereby limited resources can be used for those who will benefit most.

In summary, a policy cannot be properly assessed until quantitative answers can be given for at least these major questions:

- effectiveness and safety of the intervention;
- acceptability, response and compliance for screening intervention (long-term, where appropriate);
- total costs of preventing one critical event to medical services to participants (in physical, social, and emotional terms).

6 *The contribution to overall control of a disease may be disappointingly small* If risk were largely confined to a small and readily identified segment of the population, and if intervention confined to this group were effective, affordable, and acceptable, then a high-risk strategy would be adequate to control the problem; otherwise this approach, however appropriate to the individuals involved, cannot by itself answer a public health problem. How much of that problem it can solve will depend principally on the ways in which risk and exposure are distributed through the population.

Chapter 5

Individuals and populations

Individual variation

Motor car manufacturers try to design the best possible car to meet the requirements of a particular market and then, in theory if not always in practice, every car coming off the production line conforms to this ideal design. Humans are not like this; they are all different. Some elements of their distinctiveness may be common to a whole population. Kalahari bushmen and Eskimos, for example, are clearly built according to different designs (corresponding no doubt to the demands of their contrasting environments), but even within any one population individual people differ much more than individual motor cars—in their size, physical strength and stamina, intelligence, energy intake, patterns of behaviour and temperament, blood pressure, and a host of other personal attributes.

This is surprising. Why, after some millions of years of Darwinian selective survival, do we not all conform to an ideal height, intelligence, and athletic performance? Our variability cannot all be blamed on defects in manufacture, since near-perfect standardization is achievable when such uniformity is required. For example, humans vary but little in their basic biochemical and physiological mechanisms: we all have almost identical concentrations of sodium and potassium in the blood, delicately and accurately stabilized. Mostly, however, variability is permitted or even promoted: the attributes of individuals within a population tend to follow a rather widely dispersed 'normal' distribution, illustrated with regard to blood pressure by Fig. 2.1 (p. 42).

This variability can have major implications for health. In the Whitehall Study we found that short men (i.e. those below 5 ft 6 in (1.68 m)) were 30 per cent more likely to die in the next 18 years than their contemporaries who were tall (i.e. more than 6 ft (1.83 m)). Since the survival value is evidently not neutral, the existence of conspicuous variability suggests that there must be some compensating advantages, for the population if not for each individual. At the same time, there are also constraints on the tolerable extent of variation about the population's average.

The variation amongst individual members of a population may originate in genetic factors, or in social or behavioural forces, or in a mixture of both. The overall extent of the variation represents a balance between the forces which favour diversity and the forces which favour uniformity.

Genetic determinants of diversity

1 *Factors favouring diversity* Genetic diversity is an insurance policy against environmental change. If the environment never changed, then in time all individuals might tend towards the genetic make-up that was ideal for that environment. Such specialization could then prove disastrous in the face of migration or of climatic or other major environmental disturbance, and the capacity to survive migration would be limited. Genetic heterogeneity represents the flexibility of the species to adapt to change.

Speculatively, genetically based diversity may also be advantageous if it equips society with a range of individuals, each suited to a distinct function. There would seem to be no reason why everyone should not possess the genes for maximum intelligence. Does the fact that this is not the case imply some collective advantage?

2 *Factors limiting diversity* Those who lie at an extreme of the range are often at some disadvantage for survival and health. For example, mortality rates are greater for the very fat or the very thin, or for those with unusually high or unusually low blood pressure. The existence of genetic diversity may be advantageous, but its extent is limited by the price that must be paid for it.

Social and behavioural determinants of diversity

A genetic component contributes to variation in intelligence, body size, blood pressure, blood cholesterol, and many other characteristics affecting health and function, but in each of these there is also an environmental component. Intelligence (defined, in the only way possible, by the result of an intelligence test) is influenced by social and educational circumstances, an individual's position in the distribution curve of blood cholesterol depends on diet as well as genes, and so on.

1 *Factors favouring diversity* Within a colony of bees, all the workers are very much alike. Their tasks are few and standardized, and each individual follows the same life pattern of activity. With humans it is not so. We flourish by creativity, inventiveness, and adaptability, and that implies behavioural diversity. The Commissioners of the European Community may endeavour to impose uniform procedures and regulations on all, but this regression to the style of the beehive is resisted by the urge of humans to be individual, which means to be different.

For that large section of the world which lives in poverty there may be limited opportunity to express that diversity externally, at least with regard to diet, occupation, and housing, but economic advance reveals and enables the underlying urge to diversity. Such forces of diversification will resist any efforts to impose uniform norms of 'healthy' behaviour.

2 *Factors limiting diversity* A lady wrote to the correspondence columns of a newspaper to recount an interesting experience.
The trees in her garden provided the nesting site for a large colony of rooks. One day she observed a pair of the birds starting to build their nest at some distance from the main colony, but this independence could not be tolerated by the rest of the colony (rooks are strongly social and gregarious) and they demolished this attempt at a break-away. The couple did not give up, but persisted in a second attempt; this suffered a like fate, as did their third attempt at diversity. The day after their third effort had failed, the lady was awoken by unusual sounds from the birds. She got up and went to the window, from where she saw the rooks ranged in a circle on the grass, and in the centre of the circle was an isolated pair. After a period of agitated excitement the mob attacked the errant pair and killed them.

This gloomy tale has its counterpart in human behaviour, for although we may be strongly individual, we are also social creatures. Society feels threatened by nonconformity and resists it, sometimes harshly, and within one population only a limited range of behaviour is tolerated.

Plato wrote,

They say that Socrates commits a crime by not acknowledging gods that the city acknowledges, but some other new religion.

The result for Socrates was a fatal dose of hemlock.

Social norms rigidly constrain how we live, and individuals who transgress the limits can expect trouble. We may think that our personal life-style represents our own free choice, but that belief is often mistaken. It is hard to be a non-smoker in a smoking milieu, or vice versa, and it may be impossible to eat very differently from one's family and associates. Social norms set rigid limits on diversity, and those wishing to persuade minorities to be different from the majority would do well to remember the rooks.

Variation between populations

We owe to George Pickering (1968) the realization that the variation of personal characteristics within a population tends to form a continuous unimodal distribution. The curve may be symmetrical, or it may be skewed in the direction associated with disease. In this way blood pressure is skewed towards high levels (hypertension) whilst forced expiratory volume is skewed towards low levels (airways obstruction). The degree of skewing indicates the amount of abnormality.

Pickering was concerned only with the way in which individuals varied within a population, and he never really considered the way in which whole populations vary. For him, as for most clinical researchers, the unit of interest was the individual, not the population. Ancel Keys (1970), a physiologist, was the first to advance our thinking into new and exciting territory with his now famous chart comparing the distributions of blood cholesterol in Japan and Finland (Fig. 5.1). This simple picture carries messages of fundamental importance for preventive strategy.

Differences involve the population as a whole

It might have turned out that the high average level of blood cholesterol in Finland simply reflected the presence of many individuals

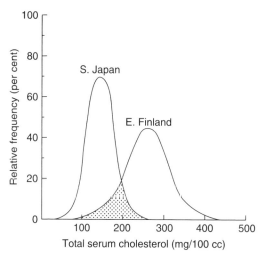

Fig. 5.1 The contrasting distributions of serum cholesterol in south Japan and eastern Finland.

with very high values, but this is not the case—the shift involves the entire population. True, the prevalence of high values (hypercholesterolaemia) is indeed high among the Finns, but if we wish to find the explanation, it will not come from studying individuals but rather from seeking some community-wide factor. This was Keys' great insight. It moves the enquiry away from clinical research (individually based) into epidemiology (population-based), and it correspondingly moves the level of preventive action from individuals to whole communities.

Having provided this eye-catching picture of cholesterol distributions in two very different countries, Keys never in fact went on to use the extensive data from his Seven Countries Study (Keys 1970) to test whether this finding could be generalized to more populations or to more variables. This was a pity, because such data are scarce. They require carefully standardized measurements to be undertaken on large samples in multiple places, and they require investigators to publish their data on whole distributions. Few investigators think in those terms! Most are interested in 'cases', and they dichotomize their data so as to report only the prevalence estimates. Others are interested in population values but only in a summary form, and so they quote means and standard deviations. Most data on distributions remain dormant in the original survey records and are lost to the world.

Our Intersalt study (Intersalt Cooperative Research Group 1988) provided us with high-quality standardized data on blood pressure and some related variables from over 10 000 men and women in 52 population samples from 32 countries. These covered the whole gamut of man's amazing range of geographical, social, and economic circumstances, from Yanomamo Indians to urban Americans, and from China to the Caribbean. The 52 samples were ranked according to the median values and then aggregated into five equal-sized clusters. Figure 5.2(a) summarizes the findings for systolic blood pressure.

The first feature is that the distributional shifts are large (more than 20 mmHg), resulting in prevalence rates for hypertension which range from zero in the Yanomamo Indians up to 33 per cent in Mississippi blacks. Such differences have major implications for public health (to be considered later).

Equally striking is the fact that, just as in Keys' example for blood cholesterol, the distributions do indeed shift as a whole. Proportionately speaking, there is as much movement at the lower part of the blood pressure range as at the upper, with the 'coefficients of variation' (ratio of standard deviation to mean) being roughly constant. (This accords with what would have been predicted from the earlier discussion of the balance between the forces of diversification and the opposing forces which restrain variation between individuals in the same society.) It follows that the explanation for the large differences in prevalence of hypertension will not be found by research into why some individuals have higher blood pressure than others, which is the subject of most current research into the causes of hypertension. We might come to understand completely why this is so, and yet still be no nearer explaining the prevalence differences, for these manifestly reflect characteristics of populations and not characteristics of individuals.

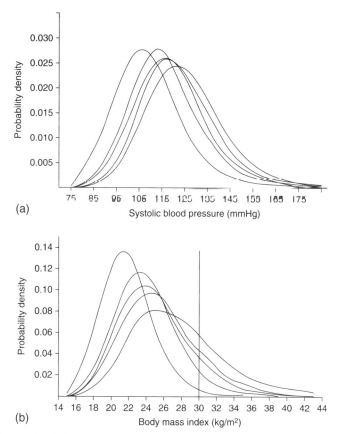

Fig. 5.2 The shifting distributions of some characteristics of five population groups of men and women aged 20–59 years derived from 52 surveys in 32 countries: (a) systolic blood pressure; (b) body mass index.

Figure 5.2(b) presents the Intersalt data for body mass index (a measure of over- or underweight). Once again we see large differences which involve the populations as a whole, with large but secondary effects on the prevalence of overweight. This time, however, the skewing of the curves towards high values increases disproportionately as we move towards the more obese populations. Evidently, the fatter the population, the more it will tolerate or support extreme variations.

In the Intersalt study we were also able to examine differences between populations in respect of other bodily measures (height, weight, heart rate) and behavioural characteristics (intakes of alcohol and salt). In each instance the differences between the 52 populations were large, and they resulted from shifting of entire distributions. (Similar examples from other fields will be considered in the next chapter.)

The 'normal' majority defines what is 'abnormal'

The word 'normal' causes a lot of confusion. Statisticians reserve its use to describe distributions with certain specific mathematical properties. However, much greater confusion results from the widespread equating of 'normal' meaning 'common' with 'normal' meaning 'healthy' or otherwise acceptable.

Taking blood cholesterol as an example, it is evident from Fig. 5.1 that what would be called 'high cholesterol' in Japan would be called 'low cholesterol' in Finland, since in every country the hospital laboratories define what they call the 'range of normal' according to what is locally common. It is easy to conclude that 'normal' results are good results.

The confusion extends to the sphere of behaviour and ethics. If most people take too little exercise (as judged by a health criterion), then this will nevertheless be considered as 'normal' behaviour and those who deviate become 'exercise freaks'. Eating or drinking 'in moderation' gets general approval, on the assumption that most people cannot be wrong. The tolerable limits of aggression are defined in relation to the local culture: what is accepted in one society may be punished in another.

In such cases the 'normal' majority has defined what is to be regarded as 'abnormal', without realizing that the standard was relative and not absolute, that it may be different at some other place or time, and that 'common' has been confused with 'healthy'.

There are, of course, strong reasons why societies should reason like that. In any social species safety lies in conformity and deviation is risky, but from the point of view of health (physical, mental, and moral) there are some glaring exceptions. Among a rural Nigerian community it had long been the custom to rub cow-dung into the umbilical stump of newborn infants despite the fact that, as a result, a third of them died from tetanus. Among modern Western communities it continues to be the custom to eat most imprudently, despite the fact that a third of the population dies of cardiovascular disease. 'Common' may be 'sick'.

The population strategy of prevention seeks a shifting of the whole risk factor distribution in a favourable direction. It faces the formidable difficulty of needing to change the majority, which means redefining what is to be regarded as normal.

Sick and healthy populations

Hippocrates, writing in the 5th century BC, advised anyone coming to a new city to make enquiries in order to assess whether it was likely to be a healthy or an unhealthy place to live, depending on its geography and water supply ('soft, hard, or salty') and on the behaviour of its inhabitants ('whether they are fond of excessive drinking and eating, and prone to indolence, or else fond of exercise and hard work').

This notion, that healthiness is a characteristic of the population as a whole and not simply of its individual members, lay dormant for a long time. It was revived and developed by Durkheim, the great French sociologist of the last century, who wrote

Each people is seen to have its own suicide rate … and its growth is in accordance with a coefficient of acceleration characteristic of each society; … and marriage, divorce, the family, religious society, the army, etc. affect it in accordance with definite laws, some of which may even be numerically expressed. Statistical data express the tendency to suicide with which each society is collectively afflicted. (Durkheim 1897)

Durkheim's argument was not simply that the suicide rate varied between countries, but that underlying these differences there were collective characteristics of whole societies. As Lukes has commented

Durkheim believed in *social reality*, a characteristic of society as a whole, and no more predictable from analysis of its individual members than the properties of water are predictable from those of water and oxygen. He tended to regard social reality as determining individual behaviour, not vice versa. (Lukes 1973)

To assert such complete independence between the characteristics of society as a whole and of its individual members is far too extreme, but in order to grasp the principles of public health one must understand that society is not merely a collection of individuals but is also a collectivity, and the behaviour and health of its individual members are profoundly influenced by its collective characteristics and social norms. Given time, these collective and societal characteristics can be changed either by the efforts of individuals, such as opinion-formers and health educators, or by the mass effects of changes in the economy, the environment, or technical developments. The efforts by individuals are only likely to be effective when they are working with the societal trends.

Collective health

Society is important in public health because it profoundly influences the lives and thus the health of individuals. Is it also important in its own right?

A population survey of depression allots a score to each individual, which is found to relate to that individual's health and functioning (p. 61). The results can also be used to calculate an average score for the whole population. What does this score imply? Since societies function collectively, may their average mood not be as important to this collective functioning as the individual score is to the individual's well-being?

There is a characteristic, 'hostility' or 'aggression', which can be measured in individuals and which relates to their individual behaviour. What does the average hostility score of a population signify? Is it the propensity to internal or international aggression? And how does it differ between populations and cultures and subcultures? What factors determine these differences? And similarly for other measures of mental and physical health.

Can such characteristics of populations be changed, or can they only be passively observed? In principle all these questions could be the subjects of research. This is largely unexplored territory, not because it cannot be studied, but because medicine has been preoccupied with concern for individuals. Therefore its importance is largely unknown, but it might be great.

Analogous questions can be asked of the physical health of populations. Fitter individuals have more energy and stamina. Would an increase in the average fitness of the population bring any corresponding benefit to societal functioning? Conversely, does a sedentary overweight unfit population suffer any collective detriment?

The main thrust of the population strategy of prevention has been to seek the ultimate benefit of individuals. It may also perhaps have a broader objective, namely to seek for healthier populations.

Chapter 6

Some implications of population change

Society seeks to distance itself from its deviants, either physically (as by segregating those with mental illness or AIDS), or by categorizing them ('hypertensives', 'depressives', 'hooligans'), or by denying responsibility for their problems (such as obesity, poverty-related illness, alcoholism, or violence). Yet in truth the deviants are simply the tail of the population's own distribution; they belong to each other and society is one, whether it likes it or not.

There now follows an explanation of these interrelations between the population and its deviants, and the health implications for the deviants of changes in the population. This will be followed by consideration of the health implications of such changes for the population as a whole.

Effects of the population average on the occurrence of deviance

It was argued in the previous chapter that within one population the range of variation between individuals is closely regulated by the balance between diversifying and unifying forces, and as a result it is to be expected that changes in the central tendency (average) of a population will be accompanied by a general shift, with the dispersion being more stable. This was illustrated by the behaviour of blood pressure and body weight in 52 centres in our Intersalt study (see Fig. 5.2, p. 93) (Intersalt Cooperative Group 1988); similar findings also apply to other health-related characteristics, including height and intakes of salt or alcohol (Rose and Day 1990). Other examples will be discussed later.

A shift in the whole distribution of population values necessarily implies an associated change in the occurrence of extreme values. The more uniform or across-the-board the shift, the closer must be

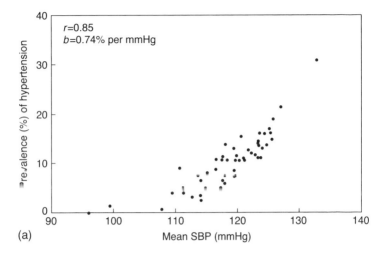

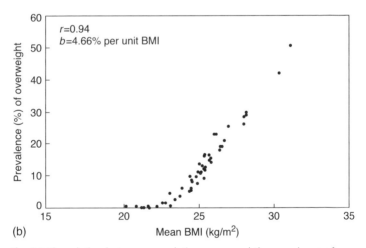

Fig. 6.1 The relation between population mean and the prevalence of deviant (high) values across 52 population samples from 32 countries (men and women aged 20–59 years): (a) systolic blood pressure (SBP); (b) body mass index (BMI);

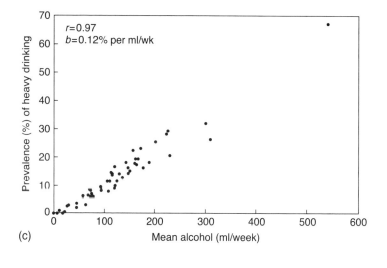

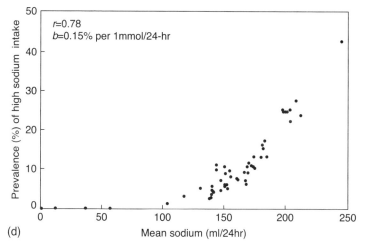

Fig. 6.1 (*Cont.*) (c) alcohol intake; (d) urinary 24-hour sodium excretion.

the correlation between population average and the prevalence of deviance. Figure 6.1 illustrates the extraordinarily close associations for four of the variables from the Intersalt study: two are physical (blood pressure and weight), and two are behavioural (intakes of sodium and alcohol). The correlation coefficients (which measure the degree of linear association, and which cannot exceed unity) range from 0.78 to 0.97. Clearly, given the average level of blood pressure in a particular population anywhere in the world, one can infer precisely the prevalence of hypertension. Similarly, the prevalence of obesity is a function of the population's average weight, the number of heavy drinkers is accurately predicted by the alcohol intake of Mr and Mrs Average, and the same is correspondingly true for salt intake.

These are factual statements on the extent to which the value for one characteristic can predict the value for another. However, the fact that the calculation of the averages includes the high (deviant) values implies an element of circular reasoning, since $a + b$ is bound to correlate with b. This can be circumvented by excluding the high values before calculating the averages; the prevalence of deviance can then be compared with these new independent values for the average in the rest of the population. The correlation coefficients are reduced, but they remain high (0.64–0.78) and statistically significant. The slopes of the relationships actually become steeper.

Such data can be used to predict the fall in the numbers of deviant individuals which would follow a general lowering of levels in the whole population. Table 6.1 shows the reductions in the population average that would achieve a 25 per cent fall in the prevalence of deviance. These effects are surprisingly strong: a reduction of one-quarter in the size of the clinical problem of hypertension and in its

Table 6.1 Reductions required in population average values (absolute and percentage change) for a predicted fall of a quarter in the number of people with 'high' values

Variable	Definition of 'high'	Required fall in population average (%)
Systolic blood pressure (mmHg)	⩾140	–4 (3%)
Body weight (kg)	⩾92*	–1 (1.25%)
Alcohol intake (ml/week)	⩾300	–20 (10%†)
Sodium intake (mmol/day)	⩾250	–40 (25%)

Based on data for UK adults aged 20–59 years (Intersalt Cooperative Research Group 1988).

* Body mass index ⩾30 kg/m², average height 1.75 m.

† Excluding abstainers.

attendant treatment might be achieved by a fall of only 3 per cent in average blood pressure; a similar reduction in the prevalence of obesity could be achieved by an average loss of 1 kg (2.2 lb) in weight, in heavy drinking if the average intake of all drinkers fell by 10 per cent, and in high salt intake by a general fall in consumption of 25 per cent. Such changes are in no way extreme or beyond reach; they only imply that most people would need to do what many in the same population are doing already.

Clinically important schistosomiasis is uncommon in the absence of heavy infestation. In instances such as this, where concern is largely confined to the heavily exposed, a general lowering of the whole exposure distribution would be particularly effective.

The implication from the above examples is simple: *moderate and achievable change by the population as a whole might greatly reduce the number of people with conspicuous problems.* Conversely, it is hard to find any examples where deviation has been suppressed and everyone conforms to the 'happy mean'. The abolition of deviance, whilst leaving the population as a whole unchanged, seems not to occur: the forces for diversity prevent it.

Examples from mental health

Among the ills with which old age threatens us, none is more dreaded than dementia. In some degree it will touch us all, and we can learn to live with it, but when severe it can destroy personal identity and dignity. The prevalence of incapacitating senile dementia varies in different communities, and much research is now devoted to searching for its causes. This research is concentrated on the causes of severe cases, with little attention to the possibility that their occurrence might reflect the mental health of the aged population as a whole (Brayne and Calloway 1988).

In the US/UK Cross-National Geriatric Community Study (Gurland *et al.* 1983) the investigators used standardized methods to compare the cognitive performance of old men in New York and London, and they reported the complete distributions of their results (Fig. 6.2). Low scores were much commoner in the New York sample: more than 20 per cent scored below 2, compared with under

15 per cent of the Londoners. However, this difference cannot be understood as long as it is viewed in isolation. As in the previous examples, we are witnessing a community-wide shift of the whole distribution of performance, involving the high (favourable) scores as much as the low. 'Why is dementia more prevalent in the New York men?' is the wrong question. The right question is, 'Why is the whole range of performance worse in this community?' The problem of demented individuals is simply an aspect of some influence which bears on the whole population. (Note that it would be offensive, and possibly even mistaken, to assume that the findings from these two samples can be generalized to their parent countries.)

In a recent study my colleague Jeremy Anderson (Anderson *et al.*, 1993) extended this approach to a more general study of mental health in the community. The Health and Lifestyle Survey (Cox *et al.* 1987) examined a random sample of 6317 British adults, and the survey included a psychiatric screening questionnaire—a modified version (the CGHQ) (Goodchild and Duncan-Jones 1985) of the 30-item General Health Questionnaire (Goldberg 1972). This questionnaire was designed for the detection

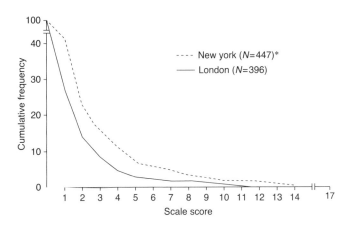

Fig. 6.2 Cumulative prevalence of scores in cognitive performance tests in old men in New York and London: the US/UK Cross-National Geriatric Community Study.

of mental illness: individuals whose scores exceed a certain cut-off value are likely to be regarded by a psychiatrist as 'cases'. The questionnaire has been validated for this purpose, and it has been extensively used in research to measure the prevalence of mental illness in the community. Because each individual examined is awarded a score, it also provides a quantitative measure of mental health and not simply an indicator of 'caseness'. This additional information has hitherto been largely ignored, and few publications include data on complete score distributions. Fortunately the data tapes from the Health and Lifestyle Survey were available for such an analysis.

The distribution of scores (Fig. 6.3) was continuous, with a single mode and no suggestion of any break between 'cases' and 'normals', implying that the commoner forms of mental illness are a quantitative and not a categorical disorder. Thirty per cent of all respondents scored above the threshold level which conventionally defines a psychiatric case: the values ranged from 20 per cent for men in the East Midlands region up to 40 per cent for women in the Northern region. (Can it really be supposed that 40 per cent of any population should see a psychiatrist?)

In Fig. 6.4 these striking differences in the prevalence of 'cases' have been related to the average scores in the various groups. The relationship is as close as in the earlier examples, with a correlation coefficient

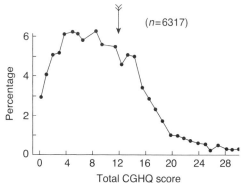

Fig. 6.3 Percentage distribution of CGHQ scores (a measure of psychiatric morbidity) in a random sample of British adults.

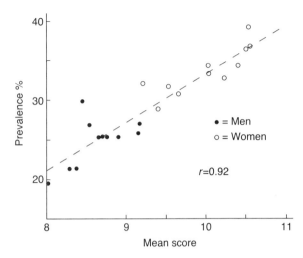

Fig. 6.4 Scatter plot of average CGHQ score against percentage prevalence of above-threshold scores according to region and sex group.

of 0.92 (falling to 0.82 if the averages are recalculated after excluding the above-threshold values). There are several important conclusions. The first is that there is a characteristic of a community considered as a whole, namely its overall mental health; this is measured by its average score. Second, this collective characteristic shows large differences between regions, between sexes, between social classes, and between income groups. These differences result from shifts of the entire distribution, with little change in the dispersion. Third, differences in the prevalence of 'mental illness' reflect the differing states of mental health of their parent communities. *The visible part of the iceberg (prevalence) is a function of its total mass (the population average).*

Psychiatrists, unlike sociologists, seem generally unaware of the existence and importance of mental health attributes of whole populations, their concern being only with sick individuals. Yet, just as even the mildest subclinical degree of depression is associated with impaired functioning of individuals, so surely the average mood or depression level of a population must influence its collective or societal functioning. It is unfortunate that its measurement and the study of its determinants have been so neglected.

The situation that has been demonstrated for results of the General Health Questionnaire, for depression scores, and for alcohol intake probably also applies to aggression. If different societies, or different periods within one society, were compared, it would most likely emerge that there is a continuum of severity and that a unimodal distribution of hostility or aggressiveness shifts up or down as a whole, for within one society there is a limited toleration of extremes, whether of passivity or aggression. If this is indeed the case, then the incidence of extreme aggression (violence and murder, vandalism, dangerous driving, cut-throat business practices) must reflect the average level of tolerance of aggression in the society as a whole, however much society and its politicians prefer to disown the violent extremists, regarding them as an isolated problem. It would be more profitable to study what determines the average hostility level of populations.

The epidemiology of the mental health of populations could lay the basis, in a way that it has not so far done, for understanding and hence perhaps controlling the mass determinants of population means, prevalence rates, and incidence rates. What determines the population's mean level of depression, alcohol intake, or tolerance of violence? What is the relation between these average levels of exposure and the associated ill health or social malfunction? What is the psychiatric counterpart of the identification and control of water pollution, which so impressively reduced the incidence of cholera?

At this point psychiatric epidemiology and psychiatric preventive action merge into social research and social policy. The two cannot exist apart (Rose 1989).

Health implications for the population as a whole

A preventive policy which focuses on high-risk individuals may offer substantial benefits for those individuals, but its potential impact on the total burden of disease in the population is often disappointing. It was seen in Chapter 4 that there were several reasons for this. In particular, most of the cases may arise among the many at lower risk rather than among the few who are at high risk, and it can be difficult to change the habits or environment of individuals if this requires them to be different from their society. What is the potential for the alternative population-based strategy? What are the theoretical implications of shifting the whole risk distribution and thereby offering a small benefit to a lot of people?

Figure 6.5 illustrates the situation schematically. We are considering the implications of exposure to some agent, such as an occupational or environmental pollutant, for which there is a graded health hazard which rises progressively with increasing levels of exposure. The diagram shows the existing distribution of the population according to exposure level: a small number of people are exposed to a large excess risk, but many are exposed to a small excess. The number of cases attributable to each level of exposure can be calculated by multiplying the corresponding excess risk (the height of the risk curve above its baseline) by the number exposed at that level. In this example most of the attributable cases will appear around the middle of the distribution because of the large numbers involved.

If a population-wide control plan is successful, then the whole distribution of exposure levels will be lowered, as indicated by the new (broken) curve. Nearly everyone now enjoys a slightly lower risk than before, and by repeating the previous calculations the new total of attributable cases can be obtained. On this basis, for example, it

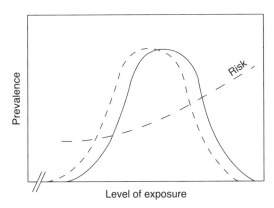

Fig. 6.5 Schematic representation of the relation between risk of disease and the distribution of different levels of exposure to a cause. The broken curve shows the new (lower) distribution of exposure after a population-wide control measure.

appears that a 5 per cent lowering of blood pressure might achieve a 30 per cent reduction in strokes (for the UK, a saving of around 75 000 strokes each year). This compares with a 15 per cent reduction in the total number of strokes if all cases of hypertension (diastolic pressure 100 mmHg or more) were detected and treated, with a consequent halving of their risk (Law *et al.* 1991*a*).

The benefits from a generalized lowering of risk come about in two ways. The first is the result of shifting high-risk individuals out of the danger zone, but the second and more important reason for the impressive potential of the population approach is the converse of the 'risk paradox' (pp. 58–59), whereby it was seen that many people exposed to a small risk may generate more disease than a few exposed to a conspicuous risk. Applied in reverse to prevention, this means that *when many people each receive a little benefit, the total benefit may be large.* (Business men nowadays are more likely to grow rich by mass sales of a cheap product than by selling a small number of Rolls Royce cars; profits depend more on the volume of sales than on the unit profit margin.)

Such calculations involve some arguable assumptions. In the first place, risk factors predict disease but they do not necessarily cause disease or predict benefit from an intervention: low income is associated with more illness, but health may not be improved by winning a large sum of money on the football pools. Further, the harm resulting from exposure may not necessarily be reversible, so that stopping smoking, for example, does not restore the lung function lost through years of inhaling irritant cigarette smoke. The estimate that a general reduction of 5 per cent in blood pressure would achieve a 30 per cent fall in the number of strokes will only be true if the relation of blood pressure to stroke is both fully causal and fully reversible. In this instance both these critical assumptions are probably true, but this will not always be so.

A third assumption relates to the characteristics of the particular community. If in another community the risk factor is less prevalent, or the associated risk is for some reason different, then the preventive potential will also be different. For example, the fact that in many countries smoking has become much less prevalent does not make it any less risky to the individual smoker but it does reduce the potential benefits from an antismoking campaign.

The sort of calculations being discussed give valid measures of the maximum population-wide benefit from a control measure, but how far that benefit is actually realizable has to be judged in each particular case by questioning the underlying assumptions.

Applications

The preventive potential of population-wide change in risk factors was first made explicit in the cardiovascular field (Rose 1981; World Health Organization 1982); its relevance to other areas is being explored only slowly, and the main (often the only) emphasis in prevention continues to rest on a high-risk strategy. In fact these concepts apply to the problems of prevention for almost every clinical speciality, as well as in occupational and environmental health and in the control of wider social problems.

All that is needed in order to explore the potential in a particular field is some knowledge of the distribution of the risk factor in the local population, together with estimates (perhaps from elsewhere) of the relation between exposure and outcome. It is then a simple matter to calculate the theoretical impact of some specified reduction in risk levels on the total burden of disease, and to assess how this overall benefit is shared among the different levels of risk exposure.

Policy-makers must then reach their opinions on how much of the potential benefit is actually realizable. This involves judgements on scientific issues (how far is the risk factor truly a cause? how reversible is the risk?) and on operational issues (how much can the risk distribution be changed? what are the resource needs and costs?). The calculations presented here indicate only what will be achievable if each of these questions can be answered optimally. In practice there will be a varying degree of shortfall.

A further element of uncertainty relates to the quality of the data, particularly those dealing with the relation of exposure to outcome. It was pointed out earlier (p. 51) that the shape of the exposure–outcome curve is critical, yet it can be difficult or often impossible to determine it. A 'sensitivity analysis' may help by indicating how far the conclusion depends on particular assumptions. The estimates that emerge are at best approximate, but despite their uncertainties they may carry major implications for policy.

Cardiovascular disease It can be said of nearly everyone in the 'developed' countries that they are more likely to die of coronary heart disease than of any other single cause. In regard to any particular age one can speak of 'low-risk' and 'high-risk' individuals, and the difference in their risks is large, but, taking a lifetime view, the difference between them is mainly that those at low risk live longer and encounter the problem later (Rose and Shipley 1990). Current preventive efforts are more likely to achieve postponement than final avoidance of disease. Even this, of course, is eminently worthwhile, the more so because life should become healthier as well as longer; coronary heart disease is now the commonest cause of shortness of breath in mid-life and later, and mild angina is widespread.

The prospect of reducing the lifetime risk of heart disease might be much better if a new generation were to grow up with a whole history of healthier habits and environment from fetal life onwards (Barker *et al.* 1989) through childhood into adult life. In many countries the diet of children, and sometimes their smoking habits also, continue to be deplorable. However, to the extent that we succeed in reducing lifetime exposure to the causes of atherosclerosis and raised blood pressure, we can hope for major gains in life expectancy, healthy life, and the lifetime risk of cardiovascular problems. The latter must necessarily imply a transfer of deaths from cardiovascular to other causes, including cancers.

In short, cardiovascular diseases are a massive public health problem in the 'developed' world, both for survival and for physical capacity. Even in those countries such as the USA, where rates have declined most, and even in those individuals with a relatively lower risk, these diseases still cause far more death and disability than any other single condition. The potential benefits from prevention are correspondingly large.

It was shown earlier (p. 85) that a high-risk preventive strategy, however promising for the individuals concerned, can make no more than a marginal impact on the total problem of coronary heart disease. This is because many people drop dead without warning, only a minority of cases occur in the high segment of the risk distribution, and screening and intervention are incompletely effective, particularly in achieving sustained control of risk factors. Thus for coronary heart disease this strategy could hardly hope to achieve much more than perhaps a 10 per cent fall in incidence, but for stroke the contribution to overall control should be substantially better, since more cases occur in the high-risk segment and treatment is more effective.

What can a population-based strategy offer? For stroke there is now strong evidence that a nation-wide moderation of salt intake would lower the whole blood pressure distribution by a few per cent. Blood pressure is closely related to the risk of stroke, and this risk is quickly and almost completely reversible. Achievable reductions in salt intake, with a corresponding lowering of blood pressure levels, should substantially reduce the prevalence of hypertension, and they should also slightly reduce the risk of stroke in the far larger numbers of people with blood pressure at or a little above the average. Taken together, these put it well within the bounds of possibility to prevent a quarter of all strokes by this measure alone (Stamler *et al.* 1989; Law *et al.* 1991*a*). Control of smoking, overweight, and high intake of alcohol would still further improve the benefit.

Similar arguments apply to the prevention of coronary heart disease. If primary prevention of raised blood pressure reduces the risk of a coronary heart attack, then lowering the blood pressure distribution by a general reduction of salt intake might achieve a fall of up to a fifth in the total number of heart attacks. For a 10 per cent fall in the average level of blood cholesterol (already achieved in some countries), one might hope in due course to see a fall of a quarter in the incidence of coronary heart disease.

Again, as with stroke, any preventive plan should be multifactorial, including anti-smoking efforts, a reduced intake of saturated fat, increased intake of polyunsaturated fatty acids, and less salt, together with improvements in the nutrition and health of mothers and small babies (p. 115). The potential public health impact of such a combined approach must be large, and this hope is being borne out by the rapid decline in fatal heart attacks which is already occurring in many communities.

Body weight Whilst half the world must struggle to get enough to eat, the other half contends with obesity and its attendant problems—cosmetic, social, and medical. Overweight is bad for health in many ways. Those in the highest fifth of the weight distribution face a doubling of their coronary risk relative to those in the lowest fifth, they are more subject to diabetes and hypertension, they become more breathless on exertion, and as they grow older they have more trouble from their joints.

In many Western countries obesity has been increasing steadily for half a century, especially in women: in Britain around a quarter of adults could now be classed as overweight, with a body mass index of 25 kg/m^2 or more. With mechanization of transport and work, both occupational and domestic, and the increased popularity of energy-dense foods, the amount of food required to balance our meagre outgoings of energy is no longer enough to satisfy the appetite. Not only has the prevalence of obvious obesity increased, but the whole distribution of weights has shifted upwards at every level (see Fig. 5.2, p. 93). This is another instance of mass change.

In considering other examples of health-related characteristics, such as blood pressure and mental health scores, the range of variation seemed to be rather rigidly constrained; the population average shifts, but the dispersion around the average remains rather constant. This is less true of body weight; when the average rises, there is a disproportionate increase in exceptional obesity. The reverse may also be true, so that weight reduction involving the upper half of the distribution may be possible without an equal degree of slimming among those who are already on the thin side of average. This would be particularly welcome because of the J-shaped relationship between body weight and total mortality (see Fig. 3.1(c), p. 52).

The excess mortality among the thinnest members of the population has never been explained. It is largely confined to older people, and it may be due to some other correlate of deprivation for which underweight is simply a marker. However, if the relationship were indeed one of cause and effect, then a lowering of the whole weight distribution (for example, Americans becoming in this respect more like Norwegians) would have little effect, for good or ill, on total mortality: the fat would gain, chiefly from fewer cardiovascular problems, but the thin would be worse off.

This anxiety may have little practical relevance, for until the world is confronted by an energy crisis people are unlikely to be willing to use their legs more and mechanized transport less, and without some general increase in energy outgoings there is small prospect of reversing the trend towards ever more obesity. Some assistance would come from a reduced consumption of fat (the most energy dense of all foods), but despite energetic health education this is not yet happening.

The ideal population policy would be a substantial and general weight reduction, omitting only those older people who are already thin. This would be expected to yield worthwhile falls in total mortality and in heart disease, diabetes, and hypertension, and gains in general physical capacity.

Birth weight (a warning against oversimplifications) The chance that a newborn baby will survive is closely related to its weight at birth. The distribution of birth weights follows an approximately 'normal' shape, though with some negative skewing, i.e. there is an excess of very small babies who suffer a particularly high mortality. In different populations the whole distribution is found to show large shifts, and distributional shifts can also occur over the course of time within one population. These shifts must presumably represent the effects on maternal health of population-wide differences in nutrition, infection, or other environmental influences. Applying the reasoning from previous sections, it might be expected that measures which controlled these influences, thereby shifting the whole birth weight distribution, might greatly reduce perinatal deaths. However, the situation is more complicated than at first appears.

The first complication is that perinatal mortality is related to birth weight in a U-shaped manner, being raised (though to a lesser degree) among large as well as small babies, and a general distributional shift that led to fewer small babies would also increase the number of large babies. The net effect on survival would then depend on the shapes and mutual relationships of the curves for weight and risk. For instance, for black American babies the present average weight more or less coincides with minimum risk, whereas for white babies the risk does not begin to increase until the birth weight is more than 0.5 kg above the average.

The distribution can be decomposed into at least two sectors (Wilcox and Russell 1986). One, constituting by far the larger part, follows a symmetrical 'normal' distribution. The other includes most of the very small babies (among whom many of the deaths occur);

this critical group does not belong in the main distribution and it is thought to relate to a different set of causes.

What are the implications for preventive policy, supposing that we knew and could influence the determinants of birth weight at a population level? In most, but not all, populations the optimum birthweight (the lowest point on the U-shaped mortality curve) is greater than the average for the predominant sector of the distribution. In such populations a rise in the average birth weight will be beneficial, although with an impact limited by the fact that many deaths occur in the minority distribution of very small babies. To reduce the size of this small but critical group calls for a different and more focused approach, since its occurrence depends on exceptional factors which operate in only a minority of mothers. It has been reported (Wynn *et al.* 1991) that dietary deficiencies are strongly correlated with birth weight in small babies but not in large babies, implying that improved maternal nutrition should have the desired effect of reducing the number of small babies whilst not increasing the number of large babies.

All medical specialists wear blinkers, which help them to concentrate. Unfortunately, patients' problems are often not confined to a single system, and in preventive medicine an intervention directed to one issue may have wider implications. Differences in birth weight, with all their consequences for infant health and survival, are intimately linked with social inequalities. In Boston, Massachusetts, mothers living in the poor eastern side of the city have smaller babies than those from the more prosperous western side. This has been related to a differing frequency of mycoplasma infection of the genital tract, and a controlled trial suggested that appropriate antibiotic treatment might eradicate the east–west difference in Bostonian birth weights (McCormack *et al.* 1987). It would of course be better still to prevent the excess of mycoplasma infections in deprived mothers; but that might involve the prevention of deprivation, and meanwhile it is something to be able to control one of its consequences.

Early development and adult health Interest in maternal and infant health has in the past been concerned simply with the short-term outcomes, measured particularly by perinatal and infant mortality. In poor countries this is still the critical problem, but in more prosperous countries a new dimension of research has been opened up by recent work suggesting that fetal and infant development may influence health throughout life.

Hints that this might be so had come from two earlier studies (Rose 1964; Forsdahl 1977) which suggested that sectors of the population with a high infant mortality would suffer an excess of cardiovascular disease in mid-life. Barker and colleagues (Barker *et al.* 1989; Barker 1991) have now shown that individuals who are small at birth are more likely to suffer from cardiovascular disease in later life or from raised blood pressure, diabetes or impaired glucose tolerance (Hales *et al.* 1991). The excess risk is less for those who grow well during the first year and greater for those who are still small when they reach their first birthday. Figure 6.6 illustrates the powerful effect of weight at 1 year on mortality from coronary heart disease; the rate for the smallest infants is about three time that for the heaviest.

These cardiovascular examples are particular instances of what could be a widely important phenomenon. During fetal and infant life a series of critical periods occur during which particular organs and tissues develop (including the brain, the pancreas, and the immune system) and physiological regulatory systems are programmed (such as those for blood pressure and metabolism), and

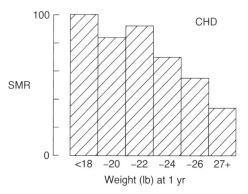

Fig. 6.6 The relation of standardized mortality ratios for coronary heart disease (CHD) in adults to previous weight at 1 year of age in 6500 males. (After Barker 1991).

what happens during these critical periods may influence the corresponding aspects of health throughout the rest of life.

It is not yet clear what external factors determine whether this organ growth and system programming go well or badly, but the strong relationship between growth in early life and adult health suggests that nutrition (or possibly infections) during pregnancy and infancy may be critically important. The next step is to identify which specific components of maternal and infant diet are important.

In order to control the major diseases of adult life, together with our disturbing social inequalities in health, it may be necessary to improve not only the nutrition and environment of adults but also the nutrition and environment of pregnant mothers and small babies.

Down syndrome Children affected by Down syndrome suffer from severe intellectual impairment, often associated with major defects of the heart or other organs, and, if they live long enough, most will develop premature Alzheimer's disease. There is no cure. Antenatal screening detects many of the affected pregnancies, which can then be aborted (if the mother so wishes).

The close relation between incidence and maternal age is shown in the first column of Table 6.2. For a young mother the risk would probably be thought negligible, but the same could not be said for elderly mothers, who face risks of up to nearly 1 per cent. The total number of pregnancies affected by Down syndrome depends on the distribution of maternal ages, and the second column of the table shows this distribution for the place and time of this particular study (Britain in the 1980s). The final column shows the (by now) familiar paradox: a large number of women exposed to a 'negligible' risk generate more trouble than the small number who are exposed to an anxious level. If special screening tests are confined to mothers aged 35 and over, then one cannot hope to identify much more than a quarter of the affected pregnancies.

How sensitive will the total incidence of Down syndrome be to a shift in the distribution of maternal ages? From the data in Table 6.2 this can readily be estimated: for each year of change in average maternal age, involving the whole distribution, the prevalence of Down syndrome births would alter by about 2 per cent. Down syndrome is

Table 6.2 Maternal age and Down syndrome (England and Wales, 1979–85)

Maternal age (year)	Birth prevalence of Down syndrome per 1000 pregnancies	Percentage of all births occurring in this group	Percentage of Down syndrome occurring in this group
Under 20	0.4	9	5
20–24	0.4	30	17
25–29	0.5	34	25
30–34	1.0	19	27
35–39	2.2	6	18
40–44	5.1	1	7
45 or over	8.1	0.1	1
All ages	0.7	100	100

responsible for about a third of the total prevalence of severe mental retardation, of which it is the single commonest cause, and changes in family planning could have important effects on its occurrence.

Alcohol Of all the threats to human health, it is alcohol which causes the widest range of injury. It shortens life, being variously held responsible for between 1 and 10 per cent of all adult deaths in industrialized countries, it shrinks the brain and impairs the intellect, it causes failure of the liver, heart, and peripheral nerves, it contributes to depression, violence, and the break-up of personal and social life, and it has been blamed for a quarter of all deaths on the road—divided about equally amongst drunk drivers, drunk pedestrians, and innocent victims (Foster *et al.* 1988). The fact that the drinking habit persists despite this toll of disasters is a measure of the personal and social pleasure which it offers (Evelyn Waugh wrote that he could never form a friendship except when drunk), reinforced in many heavy drinkers by physical addiction.

Cirrhosis mortality in France is the highest in the world, being ten times greater than that in the UK. When France was occupied during the Second World War the intake of alcohol dropped to a fraction of its previous level. Within two years deaths from cirrhosis had fallen

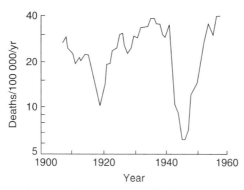

Fig. 6.7 Effects of two world wars on mortality from cirrhosis in Paris. (After Ledermann 1964.)

precipitously, almost to the British rate (Fig. 6.7). With the ending of the occupation wine became once more freely available, and within 5 years the cirrhosis rate had returned to its previous level. This episode demonstrates the dependence of health on national culture and habits, and the potential for a dramatic response when these are changed.

Interest in alcohol-associated health problems has been concentrated on the effects of sustained or heavy drinking. It requires many years of heavy drinking before there is clinically evident damage to liver, heart, or brain, and it is assumed that briefer or lighter exposure is quite safe. The experience of cirrhosis in France during the war (Fig. 6.7) is not inconsistent with this view: alcohol-related cirrhosis is a very chronic process, taking years to develop, and the apparently immediate response of mortality to the fall and subsequent rise in drinking probably means only that heavy drinking administers the *coup de grâce* to a chronically sick liver. With regard to alcohol-related road traffic accidents, outside Scandinavia (where *any* level is punishable) it is assumed that there is a critical threshold of blood alcohol level; below this level driving is supposedly unimpaired, but the driver who exceeds the critical level is punished. Social attitudes to drinking commonly reflect the same dichotomy; alcoholics are castigated but moderate drinking is accepted or even approved.

The belief that moderate drinking is harmless is unproven. In alcoholics the brain is often diminished in size, but we cannot be sure whether this represents the cumulative effect of a multitude of small injuries ('each drink kills a few neurons'), or whether neurons only perish at high levels of blood alcohol. Nor do we know the shape of the exposure–outcome curve relating drinking to the risk of a road traffic accident. This question could be resolved by comparing the distributions of blood alcohol levels in those involved in accidents and a matched sample of other road users, but such data are hard to come by. We also know rather little of the exposure–outcome curve relating blood alcohol level to social detriment. In each instance it is widely assumed that there is a threshold effect (Fig. 3.1(a), p. 52), but the alternatives (Figs 3.1(c) and 3.1(d)) have not been excluded.

The distinction is important. If a small amount of alcohol slightly impairs a driver's judgement, then the large number of drivers who have had one or two drinks would collectively incur a large excess of accidents, even though none of them individually had an obvious problem, but current policy assumes that this is not the case. Whether or not each drink kills a few more neurons might greatly influence one's feeling about moderate drinking. With regard to the social and behavioural effects, it is critically important to know at what level detriment exceeds benefit.

The overall health impact of a population change in alcohol intake would be much influenced by how it affects the moderate drinkers, but since this is uncertain (in particular, with regard to the meaning of its association with lower coronary risk), estimates must be based largely on the known effects of heavy drinking. The intimate relationship between the population's average alcohol intake and the prevalence of heavy drinking was illustrated earlier in this chapter (Fig. 6.1(c)). We were fortunate in the Intersalt study in having standardized assessments of drinking habits in so many diverse populations (52 centres in 32 countries), and we were able to show that differences in the prevalence of heavy drinking between countries involve shifts in the entire distribution of alcohol intake (Fig. 6.8). As with so many other characteristics, cultures behave coherently in their drinking habits.

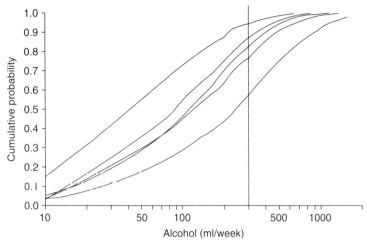

Fig. 6.8 Cumulative plots of the distribution of alcohol intake in five aggregated groups of population samples of men and women aged 20–59 years derived from standardized surveys in 32 countries.

This phenomenon was first recognized by the French mathematician Ledermann, who pointed to the obvious conclusion that the population's average intake can predict the prevalence of heavy drinking (Ledermann 1964). This assertion has aroused much controversy. The objections have been in part practical, because the survey data available to Ledermann were unstandardized and of poor quality; this problem is now substantially resolved. The more vociferous objections have been on theoretical grounds; for example, 'Ledermann's so-called single-distribution theory is not based on substantial hypothesis ... and it therefore fails to explain anything' (Skog 1985).

As a simple-minded empirical scientist, who trusts his eyes more than his reasoning, I must side with Ledermann. One may disagree about his interpretation of the phenomenon and the mechanisms by which intake distributions change, but the phenomenon itself is a fact: from the average alcohol intake of a population one can predict precisely the number of heavy drinkers. It is therefore likely to follow that changes in average consumption will lead to corresponding changes in the prevalence of alcoholism and in alcohol-related health problems.

Kreitman (1986) explored the implications of a distributional shift in alcohol consumption, as compared with the conventional 'safe limits' approach. If the latter were applied with total success, such that no one any longer exceeded 50 drinks each week (which is of course quite unachievable), then the consequent health benefits could be matched, according to Kreitman's calculations, by an across-the-board reduction in intake of 30 per cent (which is well inside the range within which populations may change over time). This specific estimate rests on some arguable assumptions, but it at least seems clear that any hope of controlling the alcohol problem depends on reducing the general level of alcohol consumption.

Osteoporosis and fractures In Britain about 50 000 people suffer a hip fracture each year. Most are elderly, 70 per cent being aged 75 or over, some die as a result of the accident, and many never recover their previous mobility. The incidence has doubled over the past 20 years, suggesting that the bones of older people have become more osteoporotic.

The determinants of osteoporosis are thought to include lack of physical exercise (bones are as strong as they commonly need to be), smoking, and perhaps calcium intake. Even a moderate intake of alcohol is associated with an increased risk of hip fracture (possibly through a greater tendency to fall). All these factors are under our control: fractured bones in the elderly are potentially preventable.

Khaw (1992) has made some interesting calculations of the potential effect on the incidence of fractures from changes in the average bone density of the population. Figure 6.9 illustrates some of the data she has used, based on an American study (Hui *et al.* 1988). The bars show the distribution of bone mass in elderly women aged 65–74 years. The line shows the steep inverse relationship between bone mass and the incidence of fractures, with an almost fourfold range of risk. Calculated in the way that by now will be familiar, the figures over the bars show the distribution of fractures. Dense bones provide almost complete protection. Khaw went on to calculate the effect on the total incidence of fractures which would be expected to follow from a general increase in bone density in the whole population, and she concluded that a 20 per cent decline in fractures would require a 12 per cent increase in average bone density. Such an increase means simply putting the clock back to where it was less

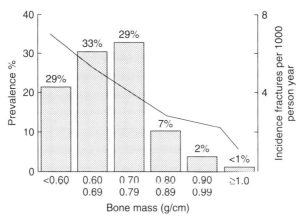

Fig. 6.9 Prevalence distribution of bone mass and its relation to the incidence of fracture (women aged 65–74). The numbers above the bars are the percentages of all fractures which occur at that level of bone mass. (Khaw 1991, based on Hui *et al.* 1988).

than a decade ago—not a big change, and one that is probably achievable by control of the recognized risk factors (Law *et al.* 1991*b*). The use of hormone replacement in women at and after the menopause could add further to the protection, but only for as long as it continues to be taken.

Occupational and environmental health Efforts to control exposure to the toxic products of industry have been prompted by concern for injured individuals (workers or local residents), particularly where a court of law may consider that the exposure was the probable cause of the injury. Someone exposed to vinyl chloride who later develops haemangiosarcoma of the liver will readily win compensation, since this exposure is a recognized cause of this rare condition. Naturally the plastics industry tries hard to avoid such a situation.

It is only individuals who can sue in the law courts: communities have no rights in law, and it is individual scandals which hit the headlines. Provided that no individuals are exposed to conspicuous risk, everyone can relax. Similarly, doctors are concerned about multiple X-rays to an individual patient rather than with the total number of X-rays. Factory chimneys are tall, emissions fall widely but thinly, and no one is at obvious risk (although tall chimneys do not, of course, reduce total emissions). Occupational physicians monitor and limit the toxic exposure of individual workers rather than the average exposure. Environmental health officers identify 'critical groups' of the most exposed people (for example, with regard to radioactivity, the most avid shell-fish eaters).

Efforts to prevent individuals from facing an unacceptable risk are praiseworthy, but are they enough? Figure 6.10 shows the radiation experience of employees of the UK Atomic Energy Authority (Beral *et al.* 1985). The bars show the distribution of their lifetime doses; the figures above the bars indicate the percentage of the total dose arising within each segment of the range (derived from the product of dose and number of workers exposed). It has been widely accepted that no employee should incur a total dose of more than 50 rems (500 millisieverts), and in general this policy has been excellently observed. It seems reassuring to note that only 8 per cent of the total dose arose in this group.

Although no one can be certain, it is widely assumed that the relation between radiation exposure and cancer is threshold free and linear. This leads to an alarming conclusion, namely that the distribution of doses in Fig. 6.10 also represents the distribution of radiation-induced cancers. The workers exposed to high doses do indeed have a personal problem, but because there are so few of them they may account for only a small part (8 per cent) of all radiation-induced cancers. Almost all the public health problem supposedly arises from the large numbers who have suffered only a small exposure and an inconspicuous personal risk. What matters for the community is the total dose. However, there is little pressure on industry to control a hazard, even though the total harm may be large, provided that no individuals face a conspicuous risk.

The critical factor underlying a national control policy should be the shape of the exposure–outcome curve at low levels of exposure. If health is damaged only by high doses, then a policy of preventing high individual exposures is sufficient, but if even low doses carry some risk then it becomes essential to consider total emissions. Where, as is often the case, the shape of the exposure–outcome curve is unknown, then the only safe policy is to keep total emissions as low as possible.

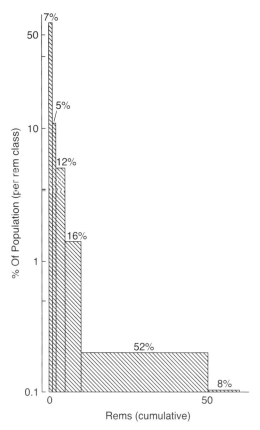

Fig. 6.10 Percentage distribution of cumulative radiation dose among employees of the UK Atomic Energy Authority.

Acceptance of the logic of this situation would have far-reaching implications in both occupational hygiene and environmental control. It is rarely possible to establish that a low level of exposure is really safe, and if that cannot be done, then the emphasis should shift from the control of conspicuous exposure to a lowering of the whole distribution by control of total emissions. Such an approach is alien to traditional reasoning; for example, in discussing the possibility that a carcinogen in bracken fern might explain the excess of stomach cancer in North Wales, a reviewer concluded that the hazard would not apply since 'bulked milk supplies and mains water would be expected to dilute any bracken-derived carcinogens to such an extent that they would no longer be a significant health risk' (Trotter 1990).

Other fields of application The examples that have been considered are only a few from a much wider range where it might be rewarding to consider the notion of a population-wide shift, either in predisposing risk factors or in the continuum of disease severity. The particular selection was guided mainly by the availability of data. Other applications worthy of exploration include intelligence, ocular pressure and glaucoma, glucose tolerance and diabetes, obstructive airways disease and asthma, nutritional deficiencies, and various aspects of communicable diseases (size of inoculum, level of immunity, sexual behaviour, and other influences on exposures). The strategy is of particular relevance to Third World countries, where resources may not permit individually based preventive measures; in particular, the need to control population growth outshadows all others (Acheson 1990).

Safety

A mass approach is inherently the only ultimate answer to the problems of a mass disease, but, however much it may offer to the community as a whole, it offers little to each participating individual (p. 47). When diphtheria immunization was introduced 40 years ago, even then roughly 600 children had to be immunized in order that one life might be saved—599 'wasted' immunizations for the one that was effective. In order to save one life from a car accident, some 400 drivers must wear their seat belts on every journey throughout their adult lives: the other 399 will take this precaution daily for 40 years to no advantage. These are the kinds of ratio that must be accepted in preventive medicine: a measure applied to many will actually benefit few. Unfortunately those few, to whom it may prove vitally important, cannot be recognized in advance.

Since the risk reduction on offer to each individual is small, then any risk from the intervention needs to be even smaller; moreover, if we are speaking of a long-term intervention, then the assurance of safety must also be long term. It is often not possible to meet these two criteria by firm scientific evidence. The follow-up period of a controlled trial does not usually exceed about 5 years, and in any case the decision to introduce a new policy cannot await a lifetime of experimental evaluation. Added to this is the problem of statistical power: in the World Health Organization clofibrate trial (Committee of Principal Investigators 1980) an excess mortality of one per 1000 treatment-years was enough to outweigh the benefits, even though the drug really did substantially reduce the incidence of heart attacks. To identify such a low-order effect requires an enormous trial, which is rarely feasible.

Addition and removal

We can usefully distinguish two kinds of preventive measure. The first consists of removing or reducing some unnatural exposure in order to restore a state of biological normality (defined as the conditions to which we are thought to be genetically adapted through our evolutionary history). Examples would be stopping smoking, avoiding severe obesity, taking regular exercise, reducing the dietary intake of saturated fat and salt, and reducing chemical contamination of foods and of the environment. Such normalizing measures can be presumed to be generally safe, and they can therefore be accepted on the basis of a reasonable presumption of benefit.

The second type of mass preventive measure is quite different, consisting not in removing a supposed cause of disease but in adding some other unnatural factor in the hope of conferring protection. This would include drugs (such as for the control of blood pressure or cholesterol), immunizations, and the use of unnatural doses of natural substances (such as high-dose folic acid for preventing neural tube defects, chlorination of water supplies, and 'natural' food additives and preservatives). For such measures there can be no prior presumption of safety, and hence the required evidence of benefit and (particularly) safety must be more stringent. This effectively rules out the use of this type of measure except where the offered benefit is rather large, i.e. in high-risk groups, or for common or serious hazards. And it should be a condition of their use that the recipients are aware of the known facts and uncertainties.

Chapter 7

The population strategy of prevention

Principles

The high-risk preventive strategy (Chapter 4) is a targeted rescue operation for vulnerable individuals. If a problem is confined to an identifiable minority and if it can be successfully controlled in isolation, then this approach is adequate (although it will need to be maintained for as long as its causes persist), but it is an inadequate response to a common disease or a widespread cause. Mass diseases and mass exposures require mass remedies. A targeted approach may assist but it cannot be sufficient.

The population strategy of prevention starts with the recognition that the occurrence of common diseases and exposures reflects the behaviour and circumstances of society as a whole. This recognition rests on sociological, moral, and medical grounds.

The sociological argument

Society exists as an entity and not only as a collection of individuals or families. Each society has its own distinctive collective characteristics, including many that influence health. These social risk factors may change, and when they do so, their distributions tend to shift as a whole, reflecting the coherent nature of society. This is the sociological basis for a population-wide approach to prevention.

The moral argument

Even though the existence of this corporate entity is a fact, it is common either to deny its existence or to reject its implications. Margaret Thatcher, when British Prime Minister, said that society does not exist, there are only individuals and families, and this view shaped her political policies. Few have the courage to state their position so explicitly, but many reveal this belief by their actions. The problems of sick minorities are considered as though their existence were independent of the rest of society. Alcoholics, drug addicts, rioters, vandals and criminals, the obese, the handicapped, the mentally ill, the poor, the homeless, the unemployed, and the hungry, whether close at hand or in the Third World—all these are seen as problem groups, different and separate from the rest of their society.

This position conveniently exonerates the majority from any blame for the deviants, and the remedy can then be to extend charity towards them or to provide special services. This is much less demanding than to admit a need for general or socio-economic change.

This prevalent view may be convenient, but it is based on a false assumption, as well as being manifestly ineffective. As illustrated repeatedly in earlier chapters, the deviant tail of 'trouble-makers' belongs to its parent distribution. The problem groups do not arise independently of the rest of society; rather, the average alcohol intake predicts the number of heavy drinkers, the average blood pressure predicts the prevalence of hypertension, the population's average mental health predicts the burden of psychiatric illness, and so on. These are facts, and they imply that the occurrence of deviance and its associated distress reflect population-wide characteristics, and hence that prevention calls for acceptance of a collective responsibility. As Dostoevsky wrote, 'We are all responsible for all'. The implications are unwelcome and most people reject them. The population strategy of prevention involves an unpopular moral choice.

The medical argument

A population strategy for prevention also rests on firm medical grounds. All major diseases show extraordinarily wide variation in their incidence rates among different populations, and often even within a single population, and most of these rates are in a state of flux, reflecting the widespread current instability of life-styles. The fact that incidence rates vary so greatly indicates at least the possibility of controlling them. Many of their underlying causes are known, relating *inter alia* to diet, housing, employment, exercise, the environment, and use of tobacco and alcohol. The objective of the population approach is to control the underlying determinants of ill health and in this way to reduce population incidence rates.

There are several reasons why effective control may need to be on a population-wide basis. The first is that many of the underlying causes are behavioural, and such activities as eating, drinking, and exercising are socially conditioned, as well as depending as much on supply factors as on personal choice. A second reason is that the incidence of many medical problems, from heart disease to hip fracture, reflects population-wide distributional shifts in the associated risk factors, and, as was shown in the previous chapter, even a small shift in the distributions may have a large effect on the number of individuals falling into the high vulnerable tail. A final justification for population-wide measures is that so often most of the attributable cases arise from among the many who fall around the middle of the distribution and are individually exposed to only a small excess risk. Thus, for instance, the total eradication of 'hypercholesterolemia' would do less to reduce fatal heart attacks than even a modest fall in the average cholesterol value of the population.

Scope

Preventive medicine is great in theory but is it being oversold in practice? It can be argued that most common diseases are potentially preventable (Doll 1982), but if one scans the list of contents of a medical textbook it becomes clear that many are still of unknown cause. They must have causes, and if those causes were known then they might be avoided, but this desirable end is not yet in sight.

Ignorance of specific causes does not in itself rule out the possibility of preventive action. One recalls the dramatic benefits to public health achieved by the reformers of the last century, whose measures to improve housing, working conditions, and sanitation antedated knowledge of bacteria and toxicology. In a similar way today one may suppose that measures to improve national nutrition and to lessen socio-economic inequalities would bring corresponding benefits to the nation's health, for even though many of the specific explanations still elude us, we know that all the major causes of ill health bear a lot more heavily on those who are socially deprived (Marmot et al. 1984).

The list of non-communicable diseases which are of known cause may be relatively short, but happily the list includes many of the commonest. Of the total loss of life-years in British adults below the age of 65, about half is attributable to just seven common disorders:

- coronary heart disease;
- road traffic accidents;
- pneumonia and bronchitis;
- lung cancer;
- breast cancer;
- suicide;
- stroke.

If knowledge now available were implemented, premature mortality from these causes could probably be halved, which would thus represent a reduction of one-quarter in the total loss through premature mortality in adults.

The realizable scope for prevention may be large and immediate, but the list of priority measures is rather short, and most of them do not greatly excite either doctors or government ministers.

Proximal and underlying causes

The immediate or 'proximal' causes of disease are the subject of medical research. They include such factors as infectious agents, dietary deficiencies (or excesses), smoking, toxic exposures, and allergens. In turn, there are the 'causes of causes', i.e. the determinants of exposure to these infections, bad diet, and other unhealthy experiences. These are a matter for social, economic, and political research.

To say that lung cancer is due to smoking is an incomplete statement and leads only to a general health education message, 'Don't smoke!' But why do people smoke? What are the causes of this cause? The answers in Western countries today are closely linked with social deprivation: smoking is rare among professional people in Britain (though not in Spain or eastern Europe), but it is widespread among manual workers, the poor, and the unemployed. When I asked Mrs Edwina Currie (then a Minister of Health) why she thought that smoking persisted in these groups of society, she replied that obviously the health education message was not getting through, and her remedy was simply that we must tell them more clearly that smoking is bad for their health! A similar view on poverty and nutrition was expressed by a minister from the Department of Social Security when he said, 'Poor people go hungry only because they buy the wrong food'. Such views are not held by those who are in closer touch with reality. Those with first-hand experience say that the association between socio-economic deprivation and an unhealthy life-style is more complex. Certainly there is an element of ignorance and lack of understanding, but a larger part is due to a much wider constellation of interlinked factors.

Underlying the proximal and more medical causes of illness are the primary determinants of these hurtful habits and experience, and these lie in the social, economic, and industrial fields. The decisions which most affect the health of the nation are not taken in government departments of health but in those of the environment, employment, education, social security, and (especially) the Treasury (Morris 1980). The population strategy of prevention operates through the medical services at the level of the proximal causes of illness, but it has to operate on a much wider base in order to confront those far more potent underlying influences, 'the causes of causes'.

This emphasis on the wider aspects of prevention does not belittle the role of the health services, but it does define it more clearly (Acheson 1990). Mortality and longevity in a nation largely reflect the incidence of its major diseases, and it is sadly difficult to demonstrate any correlation with investment in health services (Cochrane 1972). The great achievements of medical care and its recent advances are in the shortening of acute illnesses and in a most welcome relief of disability and suffering. Of course health care saves lives, but these successes are greatly outnumbered by the deaths from incurable diseases, and, for the chronic diseases, clinical success is marked more by relief of symptoms and postponement of fatal outcomes than by their cure.

Strengths of the population strategy

Three characteristics in particular are important, namely that the strategy is radical, it is powerful, and it is appropriate.

Radical

When a population is sick, it is a superficial and symptomatic response simply to treat the cases and the conspicuously vulnerable individuals; they represent the manifestation of the problem, not its roots. We need to ask why cases occur, and then to seek a remedy for their underlying determinants. Common diseases and disabilities arise because many people are exposed to these underlying causes, and a widespread problem calls for a widespread response, i.e. for a population strategy.

A population-wide approach can itself operate at either a more superficial or a more basic level. Health education is often only a superficial approach, when it seeks simply to encourage or persuade people to behave differently. A radical approach aims to remove the underlying impediments to healthier behaviour, or to control the adverse pressures. The first or medical approach is important, but only the social and political approach confronts the root causes.

Powerful

In 1777 Sir George Baker published his classic *Essay Concerning the Cause of the Endemial Colic of Devonshire*, in which he established that this common and distressing complaint was due to lead in the cider. He started his essay in this way:

A very small acquaintance with the writings of Physicians is sufficient to convince us, that much labour and ingenuity has been most unprofitably bestowed on the investigation of remote and obscure causes; while those, which are obvious and evident, *quae ante pedes sunt*, which must necessarily be acknowledged as soon as stumbled upon, have been too frequently overlooked and disregarded (Baker 1777).

Epidemiology is but a feeble tool for investigating weak causes, and it is much constrained in its study of rare diseases. Necessarily therefore, though to the advantage of public health, its principal successes relate to the major causes of common diseases, and this is where it finds its principal preventive applications. Measures to improve public health, relating as they do to such obvious and mundane matters as housing, smoking, and food, may lack the glamour of high-technology medicine, but what they lack in excitement they gain in their potential impact on health, precisely because they deal with the major causes of common diseases and disabilities.

The previous chapters reviewed some examples of the implications of shifting the whole distribution of a risk factor in a favourable direction. A 10 per cent lowering of the population's levels of blood cholesterol, such as has already been achieved in several countries, can be expected to reduce coronary heart disease by 20–30 per cent, and such a reduction of a condition that now kills one-quarter of the population would be a benefit indeed. A reduction of one-third in the nation's salt intake, again an achievable change, should reduce strokes by more than 20 per cent, and stroke is the most feared disability of the elderly. The same intervention might also reduce by up to one-half the number of people requiring drug treatment for hypertension.

Such potentially large effects of a distributional shift come about for two reasons. First, in situations where many people are exposed to some excess risk, the total benefit may be large even though each receives only a small benefit. Second, the critical level of exposure, such as the level of blood pressure requiring drug treatment, commonly occurs at a steep part of the descending limb of the distribution curve, and a small shift in the distribution can then have a surprisingly large effect on the number of people with values above the critical level.

A population-wide preventive measure may offer a disappointingly trivial benefit to individuals, but yet its cumulative benefit for the population as a whole can be unexpectedly large.

Appropriate

Personal life-style is socially conditioned. Young motorcyclists are happy to wear crash helmets if that is what their friends and role models are doing. Smokers are more likely to give up the habit if smoking brings disapproval within their section of society. Individuals are unlikely to eat very differently from the rest of their families and social circle, and the housewife buys what is readily available and attractively priced, or what is most strongly advertised. It makes little sense to expect individuals to behave differently from their peers; it is more appropriate to seek a general change in behavioural norms and in the circumstances which facilitate their adoption.

To change an established habit can be traumatic, whether it is stopping smoking, reducing salt intake, or starting to use condoms. Sometimes the trauma persists, but more often it is the change which is troublesome. The distress consequent on stopping smoking eventually passes, and established non-smokers do not continue to suffer. Food certainly tastes insipid when salt intake has just been reduced, but after a time it again tastes normal. Once society has accepted a new norm of behaviour, then to maintain the healthier habit no longer requires effort from individuals. The health education phase is an unfortunate temporary necessity, pending changes in social norms. We no longer need to be reminded to brush our teeth or to wash our hands after defecation; it has become second nature.

In developed countries the public health scene is now dominated by the chronic diseases, and control efforts have centred around the need to facilitate changes in personal life-style. This may require the collective provision of services (such as sports facilities or seat-belts in cars), or it may involve removing obstacles to free choice (such as price subsidies for unhealthy foods or lack of affordable housing), but ultimately it is up to individuals to accept or reject what is available.

The great public health reforms of the nineteenth century, which led to such dramatic improvements, were not of this kind (Acheson 1990). Actions such as the provision of clean water supplies and sanitation were undertaken for people rather than by people. They have been followed in this century by further centrally provided and regulated measures to protect or improve health, including the immunization of infants and children, fluoridation of water, control of food quality and additives, and (limited) cleaning-up of the environment.

Taken overall, the health of Western populations is vastly better now than at the start of the century. In Britain, for example, infant mortality has fallen from 138 to 9 per 1000, and life expectancy in males has risen from 48 to 72 years. Tuberculosis, diphtheria, enteric fevers, poliomyelitis, and other former infectious scourges have either disappeared or are now largely controlled. These, and many other important advances, have all been achieved largely through public health measures that were centrally provided or planned.

Successes have been fewer for those measures which call for individual co-operation, but here also there have been some notable advances. Declining rates for lung cancer and chronic bronchitis have rewarded the great health education effort to encourage non-smoking or, failing that, to prefer low-tar cigarettes, and some at least of the falling mortality from coronary heart disease can be credited to public awareness of the major risk factors. So, whether we consider interventions for people or life-style changes by people, nearly all the major improvements in national health have been due to prevention, mostly resulting from population-wide changes. Some of these changes were aimed consciously at improving health; in others the health benefit was a by-product.

There are many problems, yet unsolved, where the principles that have been so successful in the past are still relevant. There are new diseases, or diseases with a rising incidence, such as AIDS, legionnaire's disease, and other new infections, cervical cancer, hip fracture, and atopic diseases. Many of the old problems are unsolved or only partly solved, including perinatal and infant mortality rates (which are still generally much above the achievable minimum), cardiovascular diseases, mental health, and the problems of alcohol and other drugs, together with the persisting gross social class inequalities in health (Marmot *et al.* 1991); the health of the worst-off sections of the community continues to fall far short of what is demonstrably attainable.

Limitations and problems

The theory of a population approach to prevention is logically compelling, but its implementation faces some formidable problems. Does everybody need to change? Few would dispute the need to limit a dangerous occupational or environmental hazard which threatens the lives or health of identifiable individuals, but it is a quite different matter to suggest that a whole population should change its life-style or, for instance, that fluoride should be added to the water supply. Those who seek to achieve such changes must confront some controversial and anxious issues of their acceptability, feasibility, and safety.

Acceptability

In 1962 the Royal College of Physicians of London published its historic report on *Smoking and health*. The evidence seemed so overwhelmingly clear that the authors fully expected widespread agreement and a speedy change in the nation's smoking habits. They were wrong.

The report had a bad reception from the media, the government ignored it, and people went on smoking. Scientific evidence alone was ineffective.

More recently, several surveys have found little connection between what people know and what they do. Why should this be? In a sense no one can act irrationally, since there must always be reasons which determine actions, but the reasons may be complex and they are not always conscious. The smoker whose physician advises him to stop embarks on an internal weighing-up of the gains and losses, and his perceptions and valuations will be different from those of the physician. In preventive medicine the prospect of personal benefits to health provides only a weak motivation to accept a change, since it is neither immediate nor substantial, and an individual's health next year is likely to be much the same, regardless of whether that person accepts or rejects the proffered advice.

Furthermore, the population approach offers only a poor motivation for physicians. Many who embarked with enthusiasm on anti-smoking education became disheartened when they discovered that their success rate was no more than 5 or 10 per cent, for in clinical practice the expectation of results is much higher. Grateful patients are few in preventive medicine, where success is marked by a non-event. The skills required for giving behavioural advice are different and unfamiliar, and professional self-esteem is lowered by any sense of a lack of skill. Greater still is the difficulty for medical personnel to see health as an issue for the population and not merely a problem for individuals.

Feasibility

The current social, occupational, and national inequalities in health will not be much influenced by health education, for they reflect the way that societies are organized. We already know what is desirable; the obstacles to its achievement, which prevent the majority from having what some already enjoy, are substantially economic, industrial, and political.

Having already admitted that concern for future health is a poor motivator for action by individuals or even by physicians, it must now be admitted that a concern for health ranks even lower in the priorities of governments and industrial leaders, and yet without their backing little will happen, as the anti-smoking enthusiasts at the Royal College of Physicians finally came to realize.

Costs and safety

All change involves costs. The mere fact of change is a disturbance to settled routine and habits, whether in industry, social organization (road safety, health checks, etc.), or personal behaviour (eating, smoking, drinking, exercise). These costs of change are mostly temporary, but they have to be paid immediately, whereas the benefits are deferred.

Then there are the economic costs of change. Some are real additional costs, such as in providing safer facilities on the roads for pedestrians and cyclists, or in disposing of hazardous waste (British Medical Association 1991), or in financing health education. Though real these are small in relation to the health services budget. Other costs involve only a transfer of resources. For example, widespread adoption of healthier eating habits would imply major changes for agriculture and the food industry, but total expenditure on food might not be much different. Finally, there are the indirect costs of success, since reduced mortality means more survivors. The dire problems of overpopulation in the Third World came about because of successful preventive medicine, and falling death rates for coronary heart disease and lung cancer mean more old people for society to support.

Of greater medical concern than the economic costs is the issue of safety. Since a population-wide measure offers only a small benefit to each participating individual, it would be all too easy for that benefit to be wiped out by a small risk, and it may well be impossible to detect or measure such low-order but yet critical risks (pp. 54–55). A demand for certainty would paralyse all decisions.

The population-wide approach seeks to move the whole distribution of a risk factor, including its low tail, in a favourable direction. Some individuals will stand to benefit much more than others, although ideally everyone would hope to gain something (for example, by control of hazardous environmental pollution). This ideal will not be achieved if the curve relating exposure to risk is not linear, and especially if it is U- or J-shaped (p. 52). It is possible that a reduction in alcohol intake might remove a protective factor against heart attacks, and when bad housing is demolished, long-time residents suffer an upheaval in their lives. In any widespread change some people will be hurt.

The wish to see changes in a population raises many practical and ethical issues, which are the subject of the next chapter.

Chapter 8

In search of health

The Romans' ideal for personal health was *mens sana in corpore sano*—a healthy mind in a healthy body. The comparable ideal for those concerned with public health would be 'a healthy life-style in a healthy environment'. The occurrence of most diseases relates to what people eat and drink, to their daily activities, and to their physical and social environment. Some individuals are particularly susceptible to the harmful consequences of impaired circumstances, and in such cases it is appropriate to seek (or offer) a focused relief, but if either the causes or the susceptibility are widespread, then a more general change is necessary.

It is easy to say that people should follow a healthier life-style and in a better environment, but can this be achieved? Are the required policies acceptable? How effective would they be? The last of these three questions is substantially scientific, but the others are political, pragmatic, and ethical. For those who believe that politics is 'the art of the possible', policy decisions are to be guided by pragmatism, not ethics. This is close to the position reached by the late Professor Archie Cochrane, a leading advocate of randomized clinical trials. After a life-time of battles with ethics committees he finally came to the view that a trial is ethical if it is publicly acceptable. Such views are not to be taken as a dismissal of ethical considerations, but rather as a transfer of the ethical responsibility for policy decisions away from the decision-makers and over to those on the receiving end, who must judge whether it is right or wrong to give their support.

Applied to preventive medicine, as to other aspects of public policy, such a shift of responsibility away from governments and other power centres and towards the public is surely desirable, but it can only operate to the extent that the public is both informed and able to control those who determine health-related policy. At present these principles are honoured more in the breach than the observance, but there are signs of some change and we should strive to encourage them.

How do populations change?

The extraordinary instability which characterizes the incidence of so many diseases implies correspondingly large and rapid changes in our life-style and environment. In developed countries most of these changes have been very much for the better, at least in regard to health if not to other aspects of the quality of life. Absolute poverty and starvation are now uncommon, housing, water supplies, and food hygiene are greatly improved, and some of the worst excesses of industrial and environmental pollution are strictly controlled. At the same time other situations have become worse. The composition of our diet has deteriorated in some important respects, serious infectious diseases have appeared *de novo* or increased, there is more relative poverty, and there are new and more widespread kinds of damage to the environment. Either way, change is nowadays more possible than ever before, thanks to the growth of technology. The health consequences, whether gains or losses, have hitherto been more often coincidental than foreseen or planned.

Mass behavioural changes can be related to changes in *opportunity* (bicycles instead of walking, then cars instead of bicycles), in *price* (turkey, once the food of aristocrats, now the ordinary man's Christmas dinner), in *convenience* (refrigerators favour soft margarine rather than butter, and food can now be stored without salting), in *fashion* (modern Western disapproval of plumpness in women), and in *pressures* from opinion leaders and health educators (smoking in developed countries) opposed by those from manufacturers and advertisers (smoking in developing countries). Some of the ways in which these factors operate are illustrated by the example of alcohol consumption.

The alcohol example

The 'collectivity of drinking cultures', first proposed by Ledermann (1956), was confirmed by the findings from our data in the Intersalt study (Intersalt Cooperative Research Group 1988). For the first time we had access to standardized surveys of alcohol intake in a wide variety of populations (52 study groups from 32 countries). Figure 6.8 (p. 121) showed that the range of intakes was wide but that the differences reflected shifts in the entire distributions. The distributions are very skewed and the amount of skewing is itself variable, but there is no doubt about a world-wide tendency for each society to show a characteristic and coherent pattern of its drinking behaviour.

Over a period of time the drinking behaviour of a population may change. Presumably a shift occurs in the entire distribution, this being the only way to account for the cross-sectional study results in Fig 6 1 It is a mistake to expect, as Ledermann did, that such changes must follow some rigid mathematical model, but it must be accepted that most of the heavy drinkers represent simply one extreme of variation in a collective pattern of behaviour.

Discussion of the mechanism of these collective changes has emphasized the 'snowball' or 'contagion' effect. On a smaller scale this phenomenon was well demonstrated by a study of the spread of heroin addiction in the small town of Crawley, where it was found that over a 2-year period the acquisition of the habit by 58 young people could in most cases be traced back through a chain of contacts to two index cases who came from another community (de Alarcon 1969). A comparable 'contagious' spread has been proposed for alcohol (Skog 1985). Thus for some reason Mr X, a social drinker, increases his consumption. This means that when his friends visit him they are now more likely to be offered a drink and so their consumption also tends to rise, and in this way the effect works outwards through the social network. Among those affected there may be someone, perhaps with a genetic susceptibility, who is thereby carried into the category of 'heavy drinker'. In another situation the social influence might of course work in a reverse direction and lead, by changing opportunities and example, to a falling consumption.

No doubt this sort of social interaction and diffusion through the social network explains much of the mechanism by which behavioural changes come about, and it also illustrates how social pressures make it hard for individuals to behave very differently from the norm for their group, but it tells us nothing about the underlying determinants of a general change.

Price is clearly important, for if taxation is increased then consumption falls, at least for a time. Supply factors (availability of alcohol in supermarkets, licensing hours, etc.) have some effect. So too, presumably, does the massive spending on advertising, since it is unlikely that the drinks industry would be so foolish as to spend all that money if their profits were not thereby increased by more than their expenditure.

These are some of the proximal determinants of change, but we are still left wondering about the prime movers. A society's basic attitude to drinking and other social behaviours is capable of change, and when the prevailing attitude moves towards approval then all the other intermediaries tend to follow, i.e. social approval of drinking, a more permissive view of supply and licensing hours, resistance to taxation, and greater responsiveness to advertising, which in turn encourages more promotional activity.

It was shown earlier (p. 101) that the number of heavy drinkers in a population keeps in almost perfect step with the alcohol consumption of Mr and Mrs Average, and hence there seems to be no way of reducing the dire problems of alcoholism that does not involve a general reduction of intake in the population as a whole. This is hard on Mr and Mrs Average, who presumably enjoy their moderate drinking, but it is the necessary price of being members of a society rather than solitary individuals (a price that is far outweighed by the benefits of social interactions and support). Similar principles of collective response and responsibility apply to most health-related behaviours.

In Britain the societal view of drinking is generally more approving than in the USA, despite rather similar figures for current average consumption of alcohol and a much more rapid increase in Britain (+74 per cent from 1957 to 1984 in Britain compared with +34 per cent in the USA). Alcohol ranks third in British consumer expenditure, exceeded only by housing and food. For centuries the British have celebrated births, marriages, and deaths, sealed their bargains, and honoured their monarchs with a drink, and according to Gallup polls only 10 per cent of British, compared with 21 per cent of Americans, considered alcohol to be a cause of trouble in their families.

In 1984 an American federal law withdrew federal highway funds from those states which permitted the sale or consumption of alcoholic drinks to anyone under the age of 21 years. In Britain such a law would be unthinkable.

It is almost impossible to hold a rational debate about alcohol because it is embedded in our culture from the humble to the most exalted level. (*The Times*, 18 August 1981)

US policy has moved to limit both the availability and accessibility of alcoholic beverages. The British, on the other hand, despite similar public health patterns, ... have *increased* availability and accessibility in recent years. Social attitudes toward drinking, not political ideology or structure, have determined public policy. (Leichter 1991)

No doubt 'free market' ideology has also played a part. It is these underlying attitudes which enable or prevent the institution of actions for change, leaving us with the same basic questions. What determines these differences and changes in societal attitudes? Can they be influenced, or only observed? King Canute could not withstand the incoming tide, but if he had been able to wait for the tide to turn then he might have made a lot of progress.

The scientific justification for change

It needs to be better understood by the public, by policy-makers, and by medical scientists alike that we can never be certain of anything. Certainty is not a prerequisite for action. A sick patient can expect from the physician only a reasonable confidence that the diagnosis is right and that the treatment is likely to do more good than harm. Prevention should be judged in the same way, so that action may then proceed alongside continuing research and evaluation, recognizing that new evidence may mean a change of policy.

How good must the evidence be before an intervention is recommended (Rose 1990*b*)? That depends on the consequences of making the wrong decision, whether positive or negative (and also, of course, on the economic costs, but that is a different issue). For example, there is now much evidence that a reduction in national salt intake would lead to lower blood pressure and some important health benefits. The change would be cheap, safe, and only mildly and temporarily painful. There has been only one successful population-based trial (Forte *et al.* 1989), but the indirect evidence is strong and we are much more likely to do good by adopting this policy than by rejecting it.

To take a contrasting example, the situation with regard to the potent new cholesterol-lowering drugs is quite different. Experience with their predecessors warns us that unforeseen adverse effects may occur, and that these can only be identified and measured by large long-term controlled trials. It will be many years before even medium-sized trials have been completed, and no current trial has adequate power to identify important but delayed adverse effects. These drugs represent a major pharmaceutical advance, but their widespread promotion and use, outside high-risk groups, is quite wrong. The over use of drugs is a constant danger in preventive medicine and a near-inevitable consequence of mass screening.

The adequacy or otherwise of scientific evidence must be judged in the context of the particular use to which it is to be put.

Constructing the balance sheet

When a trial has shown that a new treatment or preventive measure brings a benefit, there is generally a rush to recommend its use. A recent American trial reported that a small daily dose of aspirin would reduce the incidence of myocardial infarction by 44 per cent ($P < 0.00001$) (Steering Committee of the Physicians' Health Study Research Group 1988). This sounds most impressive, but every intervention may do harm as well as good, and the mere demonstration of a benefit is never enough. There should always be a balance sheet of gains and losses, identifying and quantifying each item which needs to be taken into account, and assigning to each some measure of its uncertainty.

A convenient way to do this is to express all the items on the balance sheet in relation to one unit of the primary benefit. Table 8.1 sets out such an outline for the aspirin example. (Note that the numbers are only 'best estimates' and they have wide uncertainty limits.) When the evidence is set out in this way, two things become clear. First the data do not make the decision: we still need to think. Second, since all the items are measured in different kinds of unit, no decision is possible until someone has assigned relative values to such disparate experiences as a heart attack, survival, a stroke, and vomiting blood. These judgements on values are not scientific or medical, although

Table 8.1 Balance sheet setting out 'best estimates' of the gains and losses from taking daily aspirin to prevent myocardial infarction in middle-aged men

Gains	Losses
100 fewer myocardial infarctions	1000 person-years of taking aspirin
10 fewer deaths (all causes)	21 extra strokes
	31 extra diagnoses of peptic ulcer
	731 extra bleeding episodes (20 with transfusion)

Source: Steering Committee of the Physicians' Health Study Research Group 1988

this rarely inhibits researchers or physicians from expressing their conclusions.

Decisions for or by the recipients?

In an example such as the use of aspirin to prevent heart attacks, in theory there does not need to be any central policy decision. The treatment is offered, and individuals can then decide for themselves whether or not they wish to take it. Nothing is imposed and no one is compelled. This applies whenever the potential recipients are free to accept or reject the advice, whether it be on fluoridated toothpaste, diet, or smoking.

This freedom of choice is only effective if those concerned have access to all the relevant information and are able to understand it. In practice, access to relevant information may be difficult or impossible to obtain because those who control its supply may not wish or be able to share it fully or to present it in a neutral, value-free way. Physicians and their teams present information so as to favour what they see as the right choice, and the news media present it so as to favour their editorial policy or to make a good story.

Even when the evidence is available, it may prove difficult to understand. To distinguish a worthless study from a good one requires expertise, much evidence may be technically complicated, and a sound judgement on the overall conclusion calls for a general acquaintance with the whole field. The notion that people should make their own decisions is good, but the notion that everyone is qualified to make a scientific judgement is flawed. In practice the recipients of advice will need the help of experts to decide what the evidence means, and to that extent a decision is being taken for rather than by the recipients. However, they retain the important freedom to decide for themselves whether or not to trust the experts' conclusions.

The situation is basically different where individuals have no choice to reject a preventive measure. They can buy toothpaste with or without added fluoride, but if fluoride is added to the drinking water they can hardly avoid imbibing it. If the law says that seat belts must be worn by those sitting in the rear seats of cars, then objections may prove costly. We should expect a higher level of scientific evidence and popular acceptability for measures such as these which are imposed and not chosen by the recipients.

Social engineering versus individual freedom

Most of the fundamental statements about life and human affairs appear in the form of paradoxes. We are confronted by two irreconcilable opposites, yet both need to be accepted for both have authority.

Personal freedom is paramount, yet every attempt to change our affairs for the better must of necessity impinge on that freedom because the aim is to influence what people do. We all seek to persuade one another, whether in our families, in committees, or through political activities, and to persuade is to intrude on another's freedom. Philanthropy and freedom may be opposed.

Any policy, any kind of social engineering, puts pressure on individuals. How far should it go? Are there guidelines for acceptable interference?

Leaders and opinion-formers

History books commonly attribute to named individuals the credit or blame for events and changes. Martin Luther, it is said, started the Reformation, Napoleon led his armies against Russia, in England, Wilberforce is given credit for the end of the slave trade and Chadwick for public health reforms, and so on; right through to 'Thatcherism', history is presented as the achievements of leaders.

President Harry Truman, himself no mean leader, offered a more sober view. 'The first quality of a leader', he said, 'is to make sure that he is being followed!' If Luther, Wilberforce, Chadwick, or Thatcher had been born in a different generation, doubtless we should never have heard of them: the leadership they offered matched the needs and mood of their day, and therefore they were accepted. Similarly the North Karelia 'coronary prevention programme' is credited with leading the decline in heart disease in Finland, its success reflecting the fact that it offered the right leadership at the right time. There was widespread concern among members of the community because their death rate from heart attacks was the highest in the world, and they wanted to be told what they could do about it.

As an object dropped into a supersaturated solution will precipitate crystallization so, one supposes, leaders can precipitate social change and advances in public health but only in so far as they say the appropriate things at the appropriate time and place. There seems just now to be a strong and growing concern in the community for healthier eating, a healthier environment, and improved 'quality of life'; in consequence, political parties and leaders who espouse these causes can act effectively to focus and potentiate the trends. The tide is moving in a favourable direction, and this is a good time for King Canute to advance.

Health education

The aims of health education are to inform, to challenge, to encourage independent judgement, and (arguably) to persuade.

Information Consumer choice is free only to the extent that it is informed. Information by itself may bear surprisingly little relation to what people do, but it is the first step. People can choose what to do about the information they receive, but they are at least entitled to know as much as possible of matters that affect their health choices.

The aim of information must not be manipulation. In a scientific paper one is taught to make a rigid separation of the results (evidence) from the discussion and conclusions (opinion). So too in health education, the information should be presented objectively and with balance. This activity is quite distinct from propaganda or advertising.

A common fault is the exaggeration of certainty. Well-intentioned medical experts conceal any imperfections in the evidence and present their conclusions as though all were sure; indeed, they readily persuade themselves that this is the case. The media connive in the process by seeking simple superficially clear-cut statements, and the public generally prefers the comfort of certainty to the discomfort of balance and honesty.

Misinformation abounds, with a gross imbalance between the small resources available for health education and the huge resources devoted to promotional activities by the purely commercial interests of the food and drinks industry. Skilled and heavily funded public relations agencies can obtain coverage, in television and newspapers and even in schools, for pseudo-educational productions that are favourable to their sponsors' interests. The public needs to know who paid Dr X for his article or his television programme, and whether in the world of science he is a man of substance or a nonentity.

Leichter (1991) has drawn forcible attention to another kind of misinformation, namely, over-dramatization:

Crying wolf! … the tendency to portray each problem as the most serious health threat since the plague. Road accidents have been characterized as 'the most intractable challenge of the second half of the 20th century'; cigarette smoking as second only to 'nuclear annihilation'; and alcohol abuse as 'the major public health issue of our time.' … We will become either anaesthetised or hysterical in the face of the apocalyptic claims on behalf of a multitude of health problems, many of which originate in our own carelessness.

Information is needed not only to help people to decide what they want to do but also to help them to give effect to their wishes.

In Britain about 70 per cent of food products are manufactured and/or packaged and the principal sources of those nutrients of medical concern, viz. fat, sugar and salt, are to be found in poorly labelled package products. (James and Ralph 1992)

Continued failure to provide simple intelligible labelling of foods reflects primarily the (correct) view of certain sections of the food industry that they would lose business if members of the public knew what they were buying.

Challenge In our trial of anti-smoking counselling in civil servants (Rose *et al.* 1982) at the first interview with each man we presented a purely factual account of his situation. At its termination we urged him to think carefully about it, and to return the next week to tell us his decision. We challenged, but we did not seek to persuade nor even to advise. Almost half the men never smoked another cigarette!

To challenge is to emphasize both the importance of the issue and the individual's own responsibility for decision. It seeks to strengthen the personal right of choice, not to invade it. It is a proper and key component of health education.

Encouraging independent judgement Among the most successful of the programmes for health education in American schools are those which train children to form their own opinions on personal conduct and then to withstand, often through play-acting, any peer pressures which seek to overrule their decisions. Similarly, we like to think that the success of our smoking intervention among civil servants was due, at least in part, to replacing the traditional authoritarian approach ('You should stop smoking!') by encouraging independent judgement ('What do you really want to do?').

Persuasion? In dealing with individual patients, persuasion should probably have no part. If the patients, knowing what is involved, choose to smoke, to drink heavily, or to remain fat, then that is that; it is their choice, and one should not interfere with it.

In an ideal world the same might apply to health education in populations. The methods of the political world (propaganda) or of the commercial world (advertising and manipulation of thought) should have no place in medicine. The difficulty is the massive amount of persuasion that comes from the other side ('Drink more vodka!' 'Drive bigger and faster cars!'). Maybe freedom suffers less if it is attacked from both sides, not from one only. On that ground alone, I grudgingly allow that persuasion has some place in health education.

Such a misgiving is shared by few health educators, most of whom measure their success simply by the extent of behavioural change achieved, just as advertisers assess their success by an increase in sales of the product. Indeed, the same advertising agencies are often employed both by commercial companies and by health education agencies, and they use much the same techniques for both their masters.

Freedom of choice

Does it exist? Any form of government necessarily implies a restraint on personal liberty. Unfortunately, the alternative of anarchy would be an even greater threat to liberty, since the weak would no longer be protected from the strong. Thus attempts to regulate society ('social engineering') are not to be seen simply as attacks on personal free- dom: some freedoms are removed as the price of enhancing others, and the question in regard to any particular policy is whether or not it offers a net gain to freedom of choice.

The so-called free market system, which for a time now dominates political and economic thinking, implies freedom for wealth-generators at the price of a severe curtailment of freedom for the rest of the pop- ulation. Great efforts are made to conceal this unpalatable fact.

The European Community currently spends 60 per cent of its budget (32 billion ECUs annually) on agricultural manipulation. 'One cannot object to a shift in price policies in favour of a more healthy diet on the basis of interference with a free market dominated by consumer choice, because no such free market exists' (James and Ralph 1992). Or again, from the same authors, 'A huge amount of cat- tle and sheep fat cannot be sold directly to the consumer' (who does not want it and will not buy it) 'and therefore finds its way into the food chain in hidden form by being incorporated into meat products and other foods rich in fats'.

The whole potent system of agricultural policy and subsidies is designed for the protection of producers, not for the health of con- sumers. Free consumer choice would interfere seriously with that sys- tem, which is why the free flow of information is obstructed. Consumers are led to believe that they are being supplied with healthier fat-reduced products; they are not told that the total amount of fat produced, and surreptitiously re-entering the food chain, is much the same as before.

Socio-economic differentials are generally widening, both within countries and (even more) between the developed and the undeveloped countries. Poverty and poor education, especially in combination, imply loss of freedom and consequent health detriment. The poor must live in poor houses in poor areas. Their dietary choices tend to be worse, both from economic stringency and from lack of education. More basically, a concern for future health is crowded out by the more pressing problems of today, and self-valuation is diminished by low social status; this seems to apply as much to relative poverty as to absolute poverty. Thus people's freedom to decide their own life-style or to achieve the healthy option is already widely and severely curtailed. Health policy should aim to reduce that loss of freedom to the greatest possible extent that is not outweighed by the loss of other freedoms.

The role of governments

Much can be done by individuals themselves to improve their own health prospects, but whether or not they will actually take such action depends substantially on economic and social structures for which governments are responsible. History, alas, gives us little encouragement in this direction, for there has always been a wide gap between general principles and anything that can be regarded as practical policy. What governments exist for is not foresight (of which they are hardly capable) but pragmatic responses to challenge and crisis. Nevertheless, the nineteenth-century reformers did succeed in wresting some major progress in public health out of their responses to social and political crises, and the same could still be possible today. However, we need to be clear about our expectations.

Enforcing virtue? The first duty of government in health promotion and environmental regulation is to protect the individual's freedom of choice. Individuals who do not wish to inhale noxious fumes should not have to do so, whilst those who, for example, wish to smoke should if possible have the opportunity to do so. Neither governments nor managements have a right to impose constraints on people simply because they are believed to be good for them. If we really believe in freedom of choice, then it should be respected consistently. If they so wish, then people should be 'free to be foolish' (Leitner 1991).

This principle is not widely observed in safety legislation, which tends to be paternalistically protective (sometimes for fear of litigation).

Licensing hours for bars, crash helmets for motor cyclists, and a host of European Community regulations are enforced primarily for the promotion of virtue, though sometimes propped up by rather spurious economic arguments. The same approach lies behind the use of taxation as a means of discouraging smoking and drinking: the end may be worthy, but the means are ethically unacceptable. Virtue should not be compelled.

Ethical decisions are rarely simple, and what we need are not more rules (which inhibit judgement), but rather clear thinking and exposure of the key issues and conflicting interests. In situations where people are free to choose whether as individuals they wish to be exposed to a particular health hazard, then the choice can and should be left to individuals. Unfortunately, many situations are not so simple. If industrial plants emit pollutants, then local residents cannot help inhaling them. If workers have no reasonable alternative to employment in an unpleasant environment (including sharing an office with smokers), then individual freedom of choice cannot operate. Where exposure is collective and unavoidable, only collectively enforced control can be effective.

In Central and Eastern Europe there is heavy environmental pollution from outmoded industrial plant and processes. Cities smell—a phenomenon now uncommon in the West. There is intense pressure from both inside and outside those countries to close the offending plants as quickly as possible. One result will be increased unemployment and more economic decline, and in the end the price of a healthier environment could well be a net worsening of public health. In public and governmental perception the harm from polluted air tends to be exaggerated, whereas that from poverty is underestimated. To oversimplify an issue or to emphasize one side only can lead to a wrong decision.

Restraining the forces opposed to health It is widely accepted that governments should restrain those individuals or agencies which threaten harm to others, even though the restraint is an infringement of freedom. Criminals are locked up, drivers must be licensed and old cars must be tested, catering premises are subject to regulations and inspection, and it can be argued that the risk of transferring infection to patients may warrant the HIV testing of surgeons. The principle involved is reasonable, especially where the harm in question is serious (such as an avoidable road accident), common (food poisoning), or beyond the capacity of the recipient to avoid (HIV infection of a patient), but it must still be balanced against the costs. There is a proposal to apply to farms and cottages which provide accommodation for passing tourists the same detailed specifications for their kitchens as are judged necessary for hotels. Many of them would have to go out of business, which seems a pity.

Broadly it is a task of government to see that there is reasonable fair play. Vast expenditure to promote cigarettes, spirits, large fast cars, and poor-quality hamburgers should either be forcibly moderated or else should be counterbalanced by corresponding promotion of healthier alternatives. Heavy subsidies to farmers for producing milk and butter, but none for vegetable oils and soft margarines, creates an imbalance which distorts the freedom of consumers. This is wrong, for the outcome of government intervention on consumer choice should be to promote neutrality, not manipulation.

Enabling To enable people to make and to implement healthy choices requires information and facilities which must be centrally funded and provided. Foods must be adequately and intelligibly labelled. Advice on exercise will be frustrated unless people have ready access to sports and recreational facilities. Decent and affordable housing must be available. The unemployed require job opportunities, and young people need somewhere to go in the evenings other than pubs. If people want such things, then it is the duty of governments, central or local, to provide them.

The best predictor of infant mortality in a country is maternal education. It is through education that people learn how and where to acquire information to guide their choices, how to interpret and judge that information, and how to make and implement their choices. It is the foremost enabler of health.

Who takes the decisions?

Medical and environmental issues are often highly technical and the public cannot be expected to understand all the technicalities. This puts the experts in a powerful position, and we are in constant danger of overstepping our authority, for we are only technical experts, not experts on values or political issues. This gives the public an ambivalent attitude towards the medical experts. We are trusted because we know a lot and therefore speak with authority, and we are also mistrusted because people sense (often correctly) that we confuse our technical authority with a right to decide what is best for them.

Society, like the patient, invites health experts to give advice, both as technical experts and because our advice should be more disinterested than the powerful commercial and political pressures which they also encounter. Our responsibility is to try to offer a correct and balanced account of the scientific and technical issues, so that the public's choices can be as well-informed as possible.

Sometimes the experts are also asked, as patients ask their physicians, to advise on what should be done in the light of the evidence, and here we are in danger of overstepping our limited authority by incorporating into the recommendations our own particular set of values. Few if any expert advisory reports make that critical distinction between speaking as experts (with authority) and presenting personal views on the right responses.

Experts are also called on to advise governments, regulatory authorities, and managements. This again can create a confusion of roles. The task of a medical member of an official advisory committee is to speak as a medical expert on behalf of the public health, but the official and political members are likely to be responding to quite different pressures relating to finance, politics, and public relations. These are important and legitimate issues, but wherever they may conflict with those of public health then the medical people must be careful to keep their distance.

Political decisions are for the politicians. Their agenda is complex, and mostly hidden from public scrutiny. This is unfortunate, because often the public would give a higher priority to health than those who formulate political policies. Anything which stimulates more public information and debate on health issues is good, not just because it may lead to healthier choices by individuals but also because it earns a higher place for health issues on the political agenda. In the long run this is probably the most important achievement of health education. Those in governments who have a concern for health will be able to change those concerns into actions only to the extent that their actions are likely to win votes. In a democracy the ultimate responsibility for decisions on health policy should lie with the public. At present that does not happen.

Society cannot expect its leaders to achieve the impossible. If the public adheres to a way of life that necessarily produces much toxic waste and environmental pollution, then it cannot altogether blame industry for the problem nor expect a perfect solution, and if people choose to drive their cars faster and to drink more alcohol then there will be more deaths on the road.

The largest threat to public health: war

Modern war can kill and disable more people, more rapidly than any disease. This would be overwhelmingly true if nuclear weapons were used, but the destructive power of so-called conventional weapons is also escalating. In the wake of wars there come secondary public health disasters due to the destruction and disorganization of resources and services, and the problems of refugees and homelessness. The cost of preparations for war, and of the manufacture and trade in armaments, far exceeds all that would be needed to implement every major preventive medical programme. Against these costs there are admittedly some potential health benefits. National nutrition in Britain was improved by the wartime rationing system, and cirrhosis deaths in France fell when wine consumption perforce fell, but there is unarguably a massive negative balance overall. For anyone who is concerned to improve either world health or national health, the prevention of war and of preparations for war has to be a priority. Failure in this direction could frustrate all other efforts.

The signs of the times are not encouraging. The destructive power of weaponry grows apace. There is no evidence of any serious intention to reduce the volume of the international arms trade. Nations not yet possessing nuclear weapons are doing all they can to acquire them, and no nation which now possesses them has any plan to lose that capability.

At my last meeting before resigning as a member of the Government's Radioactive Waste Management Advisory Committee, I asked what contingency plans existed for the disposal of surplus military plutonium, if nuclear warheads were to be dismantled. The answer was 'None'. The authorities do not envisage such an eventuality.

Social and economic deprivation

The life expectancy of a female child born in southeast England is 78 years, compared with 51 years for the population of sub-Saharan Africa. Within Britain the death rates show gross inequalities: if all men experienced the same rates as professionals in the southeast, then the national mortality rate would be 37 per cent lower, but if all experienced the rates of unskilled workers in the northern region, then it would be 94 per cent higher. Nor are such massive differences confined to Britain. In New York City, where between 1980 and 1990 the incidence of tuberculosis rose by 132 per cent, the rate for blacks is 129 per 100 000 per year, compared with 10 per 100 000 per year for whites.

In our Whitehall Study of health among London civil servants we found that the best predictor of morbidity and mortality was occupational grade: over 15 years of follow-up more than 15 per cent of the messengers and timekeepers died, compared with under 5 per cent of the administrative grade. A new survey of the same population suggests that the health differential is still as wide as ever (Marmot *et al.* 1991). Much of it can be explained by measurable components of behaviour, for men in the lower grades are more likely to smoke (34 per cent, compared with only 9 per cent of administrators), their diet is worse, they take less exercise, and they complain that in their work they have less control over what they do and obtain less job satisfaction.

Striking confirmation of the importance of occupational status as a socio-economic indicator came from a study of death rates among staff of the National Health Service (Balarajan 1989), and Table 8.2 sets out some salient findings. Again one sees a near-threefold difference for total mortality between those at the top and those at the bottom, whilst for lung cancer the gap is wider still.

Regional inequalities in health are large. Like the occupational effects, they can be substantially accounted for by specific socio-economic factors (such as overcrowding, unemployment, education,

Table 8.2 Mortality ratios (England and Wales = 100), adjusted for age and sex, among health service staff

| | Standardized mortality ratio | |
	All causes	Lung cancer
Doctors	69	33
Nurses	118	96
Hospital porters	151	185

Source: Balarajan 1989

car ownership). Commenting on the health inequalities between England and Scotland, Carstairs and Morris (1989) wrote that 'the vast differences seen in the material circumstances of the two populations suggest that a large part of the excess mortality in Scotland may be attributed to the greater deprivation experienced in that country.'

Health inequalities, both occupational and regional, probably exist in all countries. They are often less obvious in developed than in 'developing' countries, in whose cities one can see affluence and extreme poverty existing side by side, but they are now being widely reported. In an American study (Comstock and Tonascia 1977) the death rate was two and a half times greater among those who had completed fewer than 10 years of education than among those who had completed 13 or more years. The authors commented that this was encouraging because 'the level of education is more easily improved by a society than income, occupation, or other indices of socio-economic status'.

Health impairment is associated with relative poverty as well as with absolute deprivation, so that inequalities are found to persist (or sometimes even increase) despite overall improvements in both the economy and health (Marmot and McDowall 1986). The sheer size of the effect seems not to be generally appreciated. It far exceeds, for example, the health consequences of environmental pollution, which, however, attracts a great deal more publicity. It is a pressing challenge to public health, nationally and internationally (Acheson 1990).

A difficulty arises, equally for researchers and for those concerned with remedial action, because socio-economic deprivation includes a whole constellation of closely interrelated factors, such as lack of money, overcrowded and substandard housing, living in a poor locality, worse education, unsatisfying work or actual unemployment, and reduced social approval and self-esteem. In turn this constellation of deprivations leads to a wide range of unhealthy behaviours, including smoking, alcohol excess, poor diet, lack of exercise, and a generally lower regard for future health. It can be hard either to isolate specific effects or to alter a specific component of the aggregate.

The way ahead

So what is the answer? Political changes which reduced economic inequalities would surely reduce also these health inequalities, with great benefit to national health overall, but at present the trends are not favourable to this fundamental remedy.

Protection from injury Smallpox was eradicated by vaccination even in countries where the conditions favouring its spread still persisted. Less dramatically, but still very significantly, other immunization campaigns have also succeeded in controlling the incidence of deprivation-related communicable diseases. Fluoridation of water supplies has reduced dental caries, even though sugar consumption remains high. These are instances of mass measures which have protected people against some of the health consequences of adverse circumstances without actually changing those circumstances. Unfortunately the list is short.

Action at the margins Within the conglomerate of factors which constitute deprivation it is possible to identify some specific components which could be tackled independently, thereby permitting some progress even though the underlying economic differentials persisted. A well-controlled trial in rural Nepal found that when capsules of vitamin A were given every 4 months to children under the age of seven, then their death rate over the next 12 months was reduced by 30 per cent (West *et al.* 1991). This is splendid. It would be quite unrealistic to recommend a better diet for all the poor of Nepal, but it is not so unimaginable that their young children should receive a cheap vitamin supplement.

More research along these lines is urgently needed, in developed as well as in developing countries, to seek for specific components of social deprivation which could be remedied at acceptable cost even though deprivation as a whole remained. Meanwhile, political effort should be focused on three broader components of deprivation, each of which profoundly influences health and where some progress would be possible even in the face of economic inequalities: these are education, housing, and unemployment.

Responsibility for health

In the age of scientific optimism it was believed that medicine had, or was soon to discover, the answers to our health problems. Thus, for example, if the President of the United States gave enough millions of dollars then cancer would be conquered. That optimism has passed (except in the popular media) and we are starting to sober up. Medicine has indeed delivered effective answers to some health problems and it has found the means to lessen the symptoms of many others, but by and large we remain with the necessity to do something about the incidence of disease, and that means a new partnership between the health-services and all those whose decisions influence the determinants of incidence (Rose *et al.* 1984; Rose 1990*c*).

The primary determinants of disease are mainly economic and social, and therefore its remedies must also be economic and social. Medicine and politics cannot and should not be kept apart.

References

Acheson, E.D. (1990). Edwin Chadwick and the world we live in. *Lancet* **336**, 1482–5.

Ackerknecht, E.H. (1970). *Therapie von den Primitiven bis zum 20. Jahrhundert.* Enke, Stuttgart.

de Alarcon, R. (1969). The spread of heroin abuse in the community. *Bull. Narc.* **21**, 17–20.

Anderson, J., Huppert, F., and Rose, G. (1993). Normality, deviance and minor psychiatric morbidity in the community. A population-based approach to General Health Questionnaire data in the Health and Lifestyle Survey. *Psychol. Med.* **23**, 475–85.

Baker, G. (1777). *An essay concerning the cause of the endemial colic of Devonshire.* J. Hughs, near Lincoln's-Inn-Fields, London.

Balarajan, R. (1989). Inequalities in health within the health sector. *Br. Med. J.* **299**, 822–5.

Barker, D.J.P. (1991). The foetal and infant origins of inequalities of health in Britain. *J. Public Health Med.* **13**, 64–8.

Barker, D.J.P., Osmond, C, Winter, P.D., Margetts, B., and Simmonds, S.J. (1989). Weight in infancy and death from ischaemic heart disease. *Lancet* **i**, 577–80.

Beral, V., Inskip, H., Fraser, P., Booth, M., Coleman, D., and Rose, G. (1985). Mortality of employees of the United Kingdom Atomic Energy Authority, 1946–1979. *Br. Med. J.* **291**, 440–7.

Brayne, C. and Calloway, P. (1988). Normal ageing, impaired cognitive function, and senile dementia of the Alzheimer's type: a continuum? *Lancet* **i**, 1265–7.

Brenner, B. (1985). Continuity between the presence and absence of the depressive syndrome. Paper presented at the 113th Annual Meeting of the American Public Health Association, Washington, DC, November 1985.

British Medical Assocation (1991). *Hazardous waste and human health.* Oxford University Press, New York.

Carstairs, V. and Morris, R. (1989). Deprivation: explaining differences in mortality between Scotland and England and Wales. *Br. Med. J.* **299**, 886–9.

Cochrane, A.L. (1972). *Effectiveness and efficiency. Random reflections on the health services.* Nuffield Provincial Hospitals Trust, London.

Committee of Principal Investigators (1980). W.H.O. cooperative trial on primary prevention of ischaemic heart disease using clofibrate to lower serum cholesterol: mortality follow-up. *Lancet* **ii**, 379–85.

Comstock, G.W. and Tonascia, J.A. (1977). Education and mortality in Washington County, Maryland. *J. Health Soc. Behav.* **18**, 54–61.

Cox, B.D., Blaxter, M., Buckle, A.C., Fenner, N.P., Golding, J.F., Gore, M., *et al.* (1987). *The health and lifestyle survey.* Health Promotion Research Trust, London.

Doll, R. (1982). *Prospects for prevention. The Harveian oration of 1982.* Royal College of Physicians, London.

Dostoevsky, F. (1927). *The Brothers Karamazov.* Vol. 2, p. 245. Dent, London.

Durkheim, E. (1897). *Le suicide: étude de sociologie.* Alcan, Paris.

Elwood, P.C. (1973). Evaluation of the clinical importance of anaemia. *Am. J. Clin. Nutr.* **26**, 958–64.

Forsdahl, A. (1977). Are poor living conditions in childhood and adolescence an important risk factor for arteriosclerotic heart disease? *Br. J. Prev. Soc. Med.* **31**, 91–5.

Forte, J.G., Miguel, J.M.P., Miguel, M.J.P., de Pádua, F., and Rose, G. (1989). Salt and blood pressure: a community trial. *J. Hum. Hyperten.* **3**, 179–84.

Foster, G.R., Dunbar, J.A., Whittet, D., and Fernando, G.C.A. (1988). Contribution of alcohol to deaths in road traffic accidents in Tayside 1982–6. *Br. Med. J.* **296**, 1430–2.

Goldberg, D.P. (1972). *The detection of psychiatric illness by questionnaire.* Oxford University Press, London.

Goodchild, M.E. and Duncan-Jones, P. (1985). Chronicity and the General Health Questionnaire. *Br. J. Psychiatry* **146**, 56–61.

Gurland, B., Copeland, J., Kuriansky, J., Kelleher, M., Sharpe, L., and Dean, L.L. (1983). *The mind and mood of aging. Mental health problems of the community elderly in New York and London.* Haworth Press, New York.

Hales, C.N., Barker, D.J.P., Clark, P.M.S., Cox, L.J., Fall, C., Osmond, C., and Winter, P.D. (1991). Fetal and infant growth and impaired glucose tolerance at age 64 years. *Br. Med. J.* **303**, 1019–22.

Hamilton, M., Pickering, G.W., Roberts, J.A.F., and Sowry, G.S.C. (1954). The aetiology of essential hypertension (1) The arterial pressure in the general population. *Clin. Sci.* **13**, 11–35.

Hart, J.T. (1990). Prevention of coronary heart disease in primary care: seven lessons from three decades. *Fam. Practice* **7**, 288–94.

Heller, R.F., Chinn, S., Tunstall-Pedoe, H.D., and Rose, G. (1984). How well can we predict coronary heart disease? Findings in the United Kingdom Heart Disease Prevention Project. *Br. Med. J.* **288**, 1409–11.

Hui, S.L., Siemenda, W., and Johnston, C.C. (1988). Age and bone mass as predictors of fracture in a prospective study. *J. Clin. Invest.* **81**, 1804–9.

Intersalt Cooperative Research Group (1988). Intersalt: an international study of electrolyte excretion and blood pressure. Results for 24 hour urinary sodium and potassium excretion. *Br. Med. J.* **297**, 319–28.

James, W.P.T. and Ralph, A. (1992). National strategies for dietary change. In *Coronary heart disease epidemiology: from aetiology to public health* (eds M. Marmot and P. Elliott). Oxford University Press, Oxford.

Keys, A. (ed.) (1970). *Coronary heart disease in seven countries.* American Heart Association Monograph 29, American Heart Association, New York.

Khaw, K.-T. and Rose, G. (1989). Cholesterol screening programmes: how much potential benefit? *Br. Med. J.* **299**, 606–7.

Kreitman, N. (1986). Alcohol consumption and the preventive paradox. *Br. J. Addic.* **81**, 353–63.

Law, M.R., Frost, C.D., and Wald, N.J. (1991*a*). III Analysis of data from trials of salt reduction. *Br. Med. J.* **302**, 819–24.

Law, M.R., Wald, N.J., and Meade, T.W. (1991*b*). Strategies for prevention of osteoporosis and hip fracture. *Br. Med. J.* **303**, 453–9.

Ledermann, S. (1956). *Alcool alcoolisme, alcoolisation,* Vol. 1. Presses Universitaires de France, Paris.

Ledermann, S. (1964). *Alcool, alcoolisme, alcoolisation. Mortalité, morbidité, accidents du travail.* Institut National d'Etudes Démographiques, Travaux, et Documents, Cahier 41, Presses Universitaries de France, Paris.

Leichter, H.M. (1991). *Free to be foolish. Politics and health promotion in the United States and Great Britain.* Princeton University Press, Princeton, NJ.

Lubin, J.H. and Gail, M.H. (1990). On power and sample size for studying features of the relative odds of disease. *Am. J. Epidemiol.* **131**, 552–66.

Lukes, S. (1973). *Emile Durkheim. His life and work: a historical and critical study.* Penguin Books, Harmondsworth.

McCormack, W.M., Rosner, B., Lee, Y.-H., Munoz, A., Charles, D., and Kass, E.H. (1987). Effects on birth weight of erythromycin treatment of pregnant women. *Obstet. Gynecol.* **69**, 202–7.

Mann, A.H. (1977). The psychological effect of a screening programme and clinical trial for hypertension upon the participants. *Psychol. Med.* **7**, 431–8.

Marmot, M.G. and McDowall, M.E. (1986). Mortality decline and widening social inequalities. *Lancet* **ii**, 274–6.

Marmot, M.G., Shipley, M.J., and Rose, G. (1984). Inequalities in death—specific explanations of a general pattern? *Lancet* **i**, 1003–6.

Marmot, M.G., Smith, G.D., Stansfield, S., Patel, C., North, F., Head, J., *et al.* (1991). Health inequalities among British civil servants: the Whitehall II study. *Lancet* **337**, 1387–93.

Martin, M.J., Hulley, S.B., Browner, W.S., Kuller, L.H., and Wentworth, D. (1986). Serum cholesterol, blood pressure, and mortality: implications from a cohort of 361 662 men. *Lancet* **ii**, 933–6.

Morris, J.N. (1980). Are health services important to the people's health? *Br. Med. J.* **i**, 167–8.

Pickering, G.W. (1968). *High blood pressure* (2nd edn). Churchill, London.

Plato *Apologia* 24 b.

Rose, G. (1964). Familial patterns in ischaemic heart disease. *Br. J. Prev. Soc. Med.* **18**, 75–80.

Rose, G. (1981). Strategy of prevention: lessons from cardiovascular disease. *Br. Med. J.* **282**, 1847–51.

Rose, G. (1985). Sick individuals and sick populations. *Int. J. Epidemiol.* **14**, 32–8.

Rose, G. (1989). The mental health of populations. In *The scope of epidemiological psychiatry* (eds P. Williams, G. Wilkinson, and K. Rawnsley), pp. 77–85. Routledge, London.

Rose, G. (1990*a*). Future of disease prevention. British perspectives on the U.S. Preventive Services Task Force Guidelines. *J. Gen. Int. Med.* **5**, S129–32.

Rose, G. (1990*b*). Doctors and the nation's health. *Ann. Med.* **22**, 297–301.

Rose, G. (1990*c*). Reflections on the changing times. *Br. Med. J.* **301**, 683–7.

Rose, G. and Colwell, L. (1992). Randomised controlled trial of anti-smoking advice: final (20 year) results. *J. Epidemiol. Commun. Health* **46**, 75–7.

Rose, G. and Day, S. (1990). The population mean predicts the number of deviant individuals. *Br. Med. J.* **301**, 1031–4.

Rose, G. and Shipley, M. (1990). Effects of coronary risk reduction on the pattern of mortality. *Lancet* **335**, 275–7.

Rose, G., Hamilton, P.J.S., Colwell, L., and Shipley, M.J. (1982). A randomised controlled trial of anti-smoking advice: 10-year results. *J. Epidemiol. Commun. Health* **36**, 102–8.

Rose, G., Ball, K., Catford, J., James, P., Lambert, D., Maryon-Davis, A., *et al.* (1984). *Coronary heart disease prevention. Plans for action.* Pitman, London.

Rosenhan, D.L. (1973). On being sane in insane places. *Science* **179**, 250–8.

Royal College of Physicians of London (1962). *Smoking and health. A report of the Royal College of Physicians of London on smoking in relation to cancer of the lung and other diseases.* Pitman Medical, London.

Skog, O.-J. (1985). The collectivity of drinking cultures: a theory of the distribution of alcohol consumption. *Br. J. Addic.* **80**, 83–99.

Stamler, J., Rose, G., Stamler, R., Elliott, P., Dyer, A., and Marmot, M. (1989). Intersalt study findings—public health and medical care implications. *Hypertension* **14**, 570–7.

Stamler, R., Stamler, J., Grimm, R., Gosch, F., Dyer, A., Berman, R., *et al.* (1984). Trial on control of hypertension by nutritional means: three-year results. *J. Hypertens.* **2**(Suppl. 3), 167–70.

Standing Medical Advisory Committee (1990). *Blood cholesterol testing. Report to the Secretary of State for Health.* Department of Health, London.

Steering Committee of the Physicians' Health Study Research Group (1988). Preliminary report: findings from the aspirin component of the ongoing physicians' health study. *New Engl. J. Med.* **318**, 262–4.

Trotter, W.R. (1990). Is bracken a health hazard? *Lancet* **336**, 1563–5.

US Preventive Services Task Force (1989). *Guide to clinical preventive services: an assessment of the effectiveness of 169 interventions.* Williams and Wilkins, Baltimore, MD.

Wald, N.J., Cuckle, H.S., Densem, J.W., Nanchahal, K., Royston, P., Chad, T., *et al.* (1988). Maternal serum screening for Down's syndrome in early pregnancy. *Br. Med. J.* **297**, 883–7.

Wessely, S., Nickson, J., and Cox, B. (1990). Symptoms of low blood pressure: a population study. *Br. Med. J.* **301**, 362–5.

West, K.P., Pokhrel, R.P., Katz, J., Leclerq, S.C., Khatry, S.K., Shrestha, S.R., *et al.* (1991). Efficacy of vitamin A in reducing preschool child mortality in Nepal. *Lancet* **338**, 67–71.

Wilcox, A.J. and Russell, I.T. (1986). Birthweight and perinatal mortality: III. Towards a new method of analysis. *Int. J. Epidemiol.* **15**, 188–96.

Wilson, J.M.G. and Jungner, G. (1968). *The principles and practice of screening for disease.* WHO Public Health Papers 34, World Health Organization, Geneva.

World Health Organization (1982). *Prevention of coronary heart disease. Report of a WHO Expert Committee.* WHO Technical Report Series 678, World Health Organization, Geneva.

World Health Organization (1989). *World Health Statistics Annual 1987.* World Health Organization, Geneva.

World Health Organization (1990). *World Health Statistics Annual 1988.* World Health Organization, Geneva.

World Health Organization European Collaborative Group (1986). European collaborative trial of multifactorial prevention of coronary heart disease: final report on the 6-year results. *Lancet* **i**, 869–72.

Wynn, A.H.A., Crawford, M.A., Doyle, W., and Wynn, S.A. (1991). Nutrition of women in anticipation of pregnancy. *Nutr. Health* **7**, 69–88.

Index